THE ULTIMATE GUIDE TO HOLISTIC LIVING

THE ULTIMATE GUIDE TO HOLISTIC LIVING

NOLAN BLACKWOOD

CONTENTS

First Printing, 2025

CHAPTER 1

Chapter 1: Introduction to Holistic Living By Nola

Holistic living isn't just about surviving—it's about thriving. It's about looking at yourself as a complete being and understanding that every part of your life is interconnected. From your relationships and nutrition to your breath and charity work, every element plays a crucial role in shaping your character. Take yoga, for instance: it can be divided into breathing exercises, postures, or both, depending on what you need at any given moment. Some practice yoga purely for its fitness benefits, while others delve deeply into yoga's spiritual aspects. Still, others use yoga to hone their control over internal and external selves. Opening your heart chakra is one such exercise, helping you become the best version of yourself by achieving balance. Performing a series of exercises, rather than individual ones, can further enhance your overall well-being.

To truly embrace holistic living, you must consider every aspect of your life. Achieving an overall sense of peace and happiness depends on the harmonious union of body and mind. The body needs a balanced diet, regular maintenance, and physical activity. Equally important, the mind needs to be challenged, but also given moments of peace and rest to function optimally. Neglecting any one of these aspects means you're not giving yourself the best chance at a fulfilling life. You must combine food, exercise, meditation, yoga, breathing exercises, grooming, relaxation, respect, and self-care in a balanced manner.

That doesn't mean you have to live like a monk to find inner peace. There are many small steps you can take to lift your spirit, connect with the earth, and fill your life with the beauty it deserves. These practices can help you become the best version of yourself and bring genuine joy into your life. By nurturing both your physical and mental well-being, you can achieve happiness and resilience. Inner tranquility provides you with the strength to navigate life's inevitable ups and downs with grace and poise.

CHAPTER 2

Chapter 2: Understanding the Mind-Body Connection

Do you see the mind and the body as two opposing forces? It's time to reconsider that perspective! The existence and health of your body, along with the emotions you feel and the actions you take in daily life, are intricately linked and influence each other profoundly.

Our mental state directly shapes how we perceive the world and how we act within it. Thoughts are not just fleeting moments—they form the core of our well-being or our suffering. Disharmony in our mental state can manifest as physical symptoms, ranging from stress-induced headaches to chronic pains. Imagine how a mind burdened by anxiety or negative thoughts may trigger behaviors and habits that, in turn, affect physical health, such as over- or undereating, poor posture, or lack of sleep.

Conversely, a balanced mental state can heal and rejuvenate the body. Just as you can mend a broken arm or recover from certain physical ailments, so too can you heal your mind. Practices like mindful meditation, affirmations, and cognitive behavioral techniques can serve as tools to fix our mental disturbances.

Every mental event has a physical correspondent—anxiety might quicken your heartbeat, while joy might bring a warm rush to your chest. When your mind is in a state of calm, this peace reverberates throughout your physical body, fostering overall well-being. Recognizing and honoring this mind-body synergy can lead to a healthier, more vibrant life. Understanding this connection leads to better stress management, improved health outcomes, and a happier, more balanced existence.

Holistic living encourages us to heal our mental wounds, just as we would our physical ones. By maintaining both realms' health, we create a harmonious existence, allowing us to live our lives to their fullest potential.

CHAPTER 3

Chapter 3: Principles of Holistic Nutrition By Nol

In holistic nutrition, the greatest emphasis is placed on creating and maintaining health by reinforcing the body's natural defense mechanisms. Central to the philosophy of natural medicine is the creation and maintenance of balance—mentally, emotionally, and physically. Health is achieved through natural means, and detoxification plays a crucial role. Practitioners of natural medicine believe in preventive measures, stressing the significance of careful screening and adhering to a lifestyle consistent with the laws of nature and the guidelines of natural hygiene. Especially in an age where disease and degeneration have become so prevalent, it is vital to ensure we are surrounded by the right physical and emotional environments to prevent and combat illness.

Your body will thrive on whole foods, regardless of personal taste preferences. The more natural, organic, and unrefined the food, the greater its nutritive value. It's essential to consume fresh organic produce whenever possible and maintain a balanced diet to support or correct your constitutional makeup. Protein sources should include nuts, seeds, and legumes, combined with a fresh variety of locally grown organic produce. Whole foods provide all essential vitamins, trace elements, and amino acids in proper balance.

Raw foods are particularly beneficial as they contain enzymes that play a crucial role in digestion. However, cooking foods above 118 degrees Fahrenheit destroys these valuable enzymes. Including raw fruits, vegetables, and nuts in your diet can significantly enhance your digestive health and overall well-being.

Cartilage from sources such as cattle tracheae or shark cartilage has gained popularity due to its success in aiding individuals with chronic arthritis, reducing inflammation, and alleviating pain in swollen joints. Chondroitin sulfates present in these sources have been instrumental in promoting joint health.

To ensure a holistic approach to nutrition, consider integrating the following principles into your daily routine:

1. **Eat Locally and Seasonally**: Choosing locally grown foods in their natural season ensures better nutrient content and supports local farmers.
2. **Balance and Moderation**: Strive for a balanced diet that includes a variety of nutrients in moderation. Avoid excess consumption of any single food group.
3. **Hydration**: Drink plenty of clean, filtered water throughout the day to support bodily functions and eliminate toxins.
4. **Mindful Eating**: Practice mindful eating by paying attention to the tastes, textures, and sensations of your food. This can improve digestion and foster a healthier relationship with food.
5. **Detoxification**: Regularly incorporate detoxifying foods and practices to cleanse your body from accumulated toxins and support liver health.

By following these principles, you'll be well on your way to a healthier, more holistic lifestyle. Embrace the natural bounty of whole foods, respect the balance between mind and body, and take proactive steps to nourish your entire being.

CHAPTER 4

Chapter 4: Physical Fitness and Holistic Wellness

Physical fitness often takes center stage when people think about holistic wellness. For many, the desire to look good acts as a powerful motivator to exercise and eat well. However, true fitness goes far beyond appearances; it encompasses strength, durability, and vitality, and it's about creating a lifestyle that supports your overall well-being.

Physical fitness, like mental and emotional wellness, integrates several practices that support a holistic lifestyle, but in a more tangible form. Consider this: your body is your temple, deserving respect and care beyond superficial aesthetics. It's not merely a vessel for prayer or a facade to show the world; it's a complex system that supports your soul and spirit as one unified entity.

Maintaining health and fitness requires a comprehensive approach, including proper nutrition, weight management, physical conditioning, regular medical check-ups, sufficient rest and relaxation, avoidance of harmful substances, effective stress management, recreation, and prudent environmental control.

To keep a holistic balance, start with these essential steps:

1. **Proper Nutrition:** A balanced diet rich in natural, unprocessed foods supplies your body with necessary nutrients. Prioritize organic produce, lean proteins, healthy fats, and whole grains to fuel your body.
2. **Weight Control:** Maintaining a healthy weight through a balanced diet and regular physical activity helps prevent chronic diseases and promotes long-term health.
3. **Physical Conditioning:** Engage in regular exercise, including a mix of cardio, strength training, and flexibility exercises. Consistent physical activity enhances cardiovascular health, builds muscle, and improves overall endurance.
4. **Regular Medical Examinations:** Routine check-ups enable early detection and prevention of potential health issues. Stay in tune with your body through regular health screenings.
5. **Rest and Relaxation:** Adequate sleep and downtime refresh your body and mind. Aim for at least 7-8 hours of sleep per night and engage in relaxation techniques, such as meditation or deep-breathing exercises.
6. **Avoidance of Harmful Drugs:** Steering clear of harmful substances, including smoking and excessive alcohol, supports your body's natural functions.
7. **Stress Management:** Employ stress-reduction strategies, like mindfulness, yoga, or spending time in nature, to maintain emotional equilibrium.
8. **Recreation:** Activities and hobbies that bring joy and satisfaction contribute to mental and emotional well-being.
9. **Environmental Control:** Minimize exposure to pollutants and toxins by creating a clean and safe living environment. This includes using natural cleaning products & reducing plastic use.

Despite the sometimes overwhelming amount of information out there, the journey to holistic wellness doesn't have to be daunting. Many people are already practicing some elements of a healthy lifestyle, even if unintentionally. It's about integrating these practices into your daily routine, making small adjustments where needed, and being mindful of your body's needs.

In an era of unprecedented pollution and stress, it might seem miraculous that our bodies continue to function. But with a commitment to making positive changes, we can start living healthier, more balanced lives right now.

CHAPTER 5

Chapter 5: Mental Health and Emotional Wellbeing

B

Chronic mental health conditions arise from a complex interplay of genetic, biological, environmental, and psychological factors. The stresses of contemporary life contribute to anxiety, depression, eating disorders, and stress-related illnesses. Work pressures, financial problems, challenging relationships, insecure living situations, dietary habits, and difficult family backgrounds can significantly affect our emotional well-being. Unresolved issues and emotional turmoil often manifest as physical symptoms, underscoring the deep connection between mental and physical health.

This interconnectedness extends beyond individual experiences to societal changes. The erosion of traditional support systems like extended families and social groups has left many individuals without the care and emotional nourishment once readily available.

Restoring and maintaining emotional health is a sensitive and personal journey, but the same holistic principles applied to physical wellness can be beneficial. If your emotional life is troubled, it's worth exploring these areas and seeking sources of help and support.

These sources might be subtle and unobtrusive yet immensely effective.

Here are some practical steps to enhance mental health and emotional well-being:

1. **Acknowledging Feelings:** Understand that it's okay to feel overwhelmed or distressed. Recognizing and accepting your emotions is the first step toward healing.
2. **Seeking Support:** Don't hesitate to reach out to friends, family, or professional counselors. Support networks can provide the care and emotional nourishment you need.
3. **Mindfulness and Meditation:** Practicing mindfulness and meditation can center your thoughts and help you reconnect with your inner self. These practices reduce stress and promote a sense of peace.
4. **Healthy Lifestyle Choices:** Engage in activities that enhance your overall well-being. Regular exercise, balanced nutrition, and ample sleep create a strong foundation for emotional stability.
5. **Creative Outlets:** Channel your emotions through creative pursuits such as writing, painting, music, or any other form of artistic expression. Creativity offers a therapeutic release.
6. **Limiting Technology:** Reduce screen time and limit exposure to social media. Constant online engagement can heighten anxiety and disrupt emotional balance.
7. **Professional Help:** Consulting therapists, psychologists, or other mental health professionals can provide tailored interventions and therapeutic strategies.
8. **Community Involvement:** Becoming part of a community or social group that shares similar interests or experiences can provide a sense of belonging and reduce feelings of isolation.

9. **Self-Compassion:** Treat yourself with the kindness and understanding you would offer to a friend. Self-compassion helps reduce negative self-talk and promotes emotional resilience.

By actively working on these areas, you can create a supportive environment to foster mental and emotional well-being. The journey to restoring emotional health can be challenging, but the rewards are truly life-enhancing. Emotional health and happiness are integral components of a holistic lifestyle, essential for anyone seeking a fulfilling and harmonious existence.

CHAPTER 6

Chapter 6: Spirituality and Holistic Living By Nol

Holistic living is deeply interconnected with our spiritual selves. Honoring our true spirit shapes our worldview, colors our intentions and actions, and forms the foundation of weaving our lives into something warm and meaningful. If our worldviews don't include justice, compassion, and equality, our spirituality remains underrealized. True spirituality transcends mere beliefs—it defines our purpose, illuminates our values, and connects us to every relationship in our lives.

Our understanding of the divine deeply influences our values, perspectives on money, personas, decisions, worldviews, and life goals. The intricate dance between faith and daily life is full of unique complexities, differing from person to person. To honor our spirituality, we must be open to seeing each person as an expression of the divine. This means ensuring that our beliefs do not marginalize anyone and making sure our materialism and desires do not obstruct others from living meaningful lives. By continually striving toward the manifestation of our divine potential, we create a harmonious existence.

Here are some ways to integrate spirituality into holistic living:

1. **Mindful Presence:** Practice being fully present in each moment. This awareness helps you connect more deeply with yourself and others, enriching your spiritual journey.
2. **Daily Reflection:** Set aside time each day for reflection. Whether through meditation, prayer, journaling, or quiet contemplation, introspective practices can deepen your understanding of your spiritual path.
3. **Acts of Kindness:** Engage in acts of kindness and service. Helping others not only benefits them but also brings you closer to your spiritual essence.
4. **Purposeful Living:** Align your actions with your values and purpose. Make decisions that reflect your true self and contribute positively to the world around you.
5. **Interconnectedness:** Recognize the interconnectedness of all beings. This perspective fosters empathy and compassion, essential qualities for holistic living.
6. **Spiritual Community:** Join or create a community that supports your spiritual growth. Sharing your journey with like-minded individuals can provide encouragement and deeper insights.
7. **Nature Connection:** Spend time in nature to reconnect with the earth and find inspiration in the beauty of the natural world. Nature can be a powerful source of spiritual renewal.
8. **Gratitude Practice:** Cultivate a habit of gratitude. Recognizing and appreciating the blessings in your life can shift your mindset and enhance your spiritual well-being.

By integrating these practices into your daily life, you honor your spirituality and create a path toward a more meaningful and fulfilling existence. Spirituality isn't just about personal enlightenment—it's about fostering a world that reflects divine love, justice, and compassion. Through conscious choices and actions, you can contribute to a collective spirituality that uplifts and unites.

CHAPTER 7

Chapter 7: Holistic Approaches to Stress Managemen

Combating and managing stress is an essential component of holistic living. When the mind is at peace and in balance, the body becomes more capable of resisting disease, naturally gravitating toward a state of stillness and healing. Conversely, when the body is imbalanced due to improper care and fatigue, the mind struggles to find rest.

Inside every human being lies a deep reservoir of peace and happiness. Within the framework of holistic living, when layers of stress are peeled away, these qualities emerge. Rather than merely addressing the symptoms of stress, holistic stress relief focuses on the root cause, ensuring that the mind, body, and spirit are in harmony.

Stress is a universal experience—everyone encounters it to varying degrees at different times in their life. However, it's common to either dismiss or overlook the signs of stress. Physiological changes occur in our bodies when we are under stress, and prolonged exposure can weaken the immune system, making us more susceptible to illness.

Several holistic interventions can be incorporated into your daily routine to manage stress effectively:

1. **Yoga**: Practicing yoga combines physical postures, breathing techniques, and meditation to help relieve stress and promote relaxation. The emphasis on mindful movement and deep breathing facilitates a state of inner calm.
2. **Mind-Body Exercises**: Activities such as tai chi and qigong blend gentle physical exercise, breathing methods, and meditation, enhancing the connection between the mind and body while reducing stress.
3. **Aromatherapy**: Utilizing essential oils like lavender, chamomile, and sandalwood can create a calming atmosphere. Diffusing these oils or incorporating them into massage routines can help alleviate stress.
4. **Energy-Based Approaches**: Techniques like Reiki and acupuncture are designed to balance the body's energy flow, promote relaxation, and reduce stress.
5. **Burnout Prevention and Management**: Recognizing the signs of burnout is crucial for maintaining a balanced life. Tips for preventing burnout include setting realistic goals, taking regular breaks, practicing self-care, and seeking support when needed.
6. **Meditation and Mindfulness**: Regular meditation practice cultivates mindfulness, which enhances our ability to remain present and manage stress more effectively. Techniques such as guided meditation or focused attention on breathing can be particularly beneficial.
7. **Nature Therapy**: Spending time in nature has a grounding effect and can reduce stress levels. Activities such as hiking,

gardening, or simply taking a walk in a park can help you reconnect with the natural world.

8. **Creative Expression**: Engaging in creative activities like painting, writing, or music allows for emotional release and stress reduction.

Implementing these holistic practices can significantly enhance your ability to cope with stress. By addressing the root causes and promoting harmony between the mind, body, and spirit, you'll pave the way for a more tranquil and balanced life.

CHAPTER 8

Chapter 8: The Importance of Sleep in Holistic Hea

Obtaining restful and consistent nighttime sleep is crucial to enjoying vibrant holistic health. As illustrated in the appendix chapter called "Model of Five Circles," sleep is shown as the fifth circle that connects all the others, symbolizing how sleep underpins and drives every other aspect of holistic living.

High-quality, continuous, and adequate sleep is essential for regeneration on multiple levels:

- **Physically**: During deep sleep, our bodies release melatonin, a precious sleep-inducing hormone that facilitates physical regeneration and repair.
- **Mentally**: Adequate sleep helps regulate appetite hormones such as ghrelin and leptin, contributing to better mental health and weight management.
- **Spiritually**: Deep sleep supports mental and spiritual recovery, providing a foundation for emotional equilibrium and inner peace.

However, many people struggle to achieve a solid night's sleep, leading to negative effects on their energy levels and overall well-being. This lack of proper rest can result in difficulties participating in a meaningful daily life, as fatigue and irritability set in.

Here are some holistic tips to improve sleep quality:

1. **Establish a Sleep Routine**: Consistency is key. Go to bed and wake up at the same time every day, even on weekends. This helps regulate your body's internal clock.
2. **Create a Relaxing Bedtime Ritual**: Develop a pre-sleep routine that includes activities that calm your mind and body. Reading, taking a warm bath, or practicing gentle yoga can signal to your body that it's time to wind down.
3. **Optimize Your Sleep Environment**: Ensure your bedroom is conducive to sleep. Keep it cool, dark, and quiet. Consider using blackout curtains, earplugs, or white noise machines.
4. **Limit Screen Time Before Bed**: The blue light emitted by phones, tablets, and computers can interfere with melatonin production. Try to shut off screens at least an hour before bedtime.
5. **Mind Your Diet**: Avoid heavy meals, caffeine, and alcohol close to bedtime. These can disrupt your sleep cycle and cause discomfort.
6. **Stay Active**: Regular physical activity can help you fall asleep faster and enjoy deeper sleep. However, avoid vigorous exercise close to bedtime as it may have the opposite effect.
7. **Practice Mindfulness and Meditation**: Techniques like mindfulness meditation can reduce stress and promote a peaceful mind ready for rest.
8. **Consider Natural Sleep Aids**: Some people find that natural supplements, such as melatonin or valerian root, can aid

in achieving restful sleep. Always consult with a healthcare provider before starting any new supplements.

By incorporating these practices, you can improve your sleep quality, leading to better physical, mental, and spiritual health. Sleep is not just a passive state but an active process of restoration and rejuvenation that plays a vital role in holistic living.

CHAPTER 9

Chapter 9: Environmental Wellness and Sustainable

For many today, it's important that their behaviors support and protect the environment. As scientific evidence accumulates, we better understand the long-term effects of human behaviors on the environment and recognize the need for consistent actions to sustain our natural resources for future generations. Living in a way that respects the unique needs of the environment and being mindful of future generations is a cornerstone of environmental wellness and responsibility.

Environmental wellness encompasses living in a way that minimizes harmful effects on our surroundings. This practice helps develop healthy habits that support personal wellness and contribute to a healthier planet. Initiating this process within your own living environment is crucial, setting an example for others by adopting sustainable practices.

Here are some practical steps for fostering environmental wellness:

1. **Reduce, Reuse, Recycle**: This fundamental principle helps minimize waste and conserve natural resources. Make it a habit to reduce consumption, repurpose items, and recycle whenever possible.
2. **Energy Efficiency**: Save energy by using energy-efficient appliances and light bulbs, unplugging electronics when not in use, and utilizing natural light. Consider transitioning to renewable energy sources like solar or wind power.
3. **Water Conservation**: Use water-saving fixtures, fix leaks promptly, and be mindful of water usage. Simple actions like turning off the tap while brushing teeth or taking shorter showers can make a significant impact.
4. **Sustainable Transportation**: Opt for walking, cycling, or public transportation when possible. If you drive, consider carpooling or using fuel-efficient vehicles.
5. **Organic and Local Foods**: Support local farmers by purchasing organic and locally grown produce. This reduces the carbon footprint associated with long-distance transport and promotes healthier eating.
6. **Eco-Friendly Products**: Choose products made from sustainable materials and those free from harmful chemicals. Look for certifications like Fair Trade, USDA Organic, and Eco-Cert.
7. **Green Spaces**: Incorporate plants into your living spaces and support community gardens and green spaces. Plants not only improve air quality but also provide a sense of tranquility and connection to nature.
8. **Education and Advocacy**: Stay informed about environmental issues and advocate for policies that protect the environment. Share your knowledge and encourage others to adopt sustainable practices.

Incorporating these steps into your daily life can transform your lifestyle into one that prioritizes environmental wellness. The desire to foster stewardship and personal responsibility extends beyond mere marketing and into education and outreach. By championing sustainable living and teaching the next generation the importance of environmental care, we pave the way for a healthier planet.

Holistic health means that your children are less likely to face serious problems from environmental concerns. By adopting sustainable practices now, you create a safer, healthier world for future generations.

CHAPTER 10

Chapter 10: Holistic Practices from Around the Wor

Yoga, an ancient practice over five thousand years old, offers a union of the body, mind, and spirit. This science of self-realization remains valid today. Traditionally, Akhanda yoga's great value lies in practicing Asana within the context of Pranayama (breath control), Bandhas (energy locks), and Mudras (gestures), as well as Kriyas (cleansing techniques) and Dhyana (meditation). This holistic system promotes health and spiritual enlightenment. One dictionary definition of Yoga is "joining the ego with the divine nature of all." Akhanda yoga supports this by providing balance, strengthening the body, soothing the mind, and fostering spiritual awareness.

Aromatherapy is a specialized massage technique using pure, therapeutic essential oils derived from herbs, flowers, and medicinal plants. The oils are applied topically to each foot and the corresponding spine reflex points from the nape of the neck down to the big toe. With custom strokes, the oils are massaged into the feet and spine reflexes. These essential oil molecules are small enough to cross both the blood-brain and placenta barriers, reaching the cellular level in seconds. The oils pass through the lipid bilayers of cells, carrying oxygen, nutrients, and other needed molecules into the cells while expelling waste through the lungs, kidneys, and urinary bladder.

Beyond yoga and aromatherapy, several holistic practices worldwide contribute to overall well-being. Here are a few notable ones:

1. **Ayurveda (India)**: Known as the "science of life," Ayurveda emphasizes balance in the body, mind, and spirit through diet, herbal treatments, and yogic breathing.
2. **Traditional Chinese Medicine (China)**: This includes acupuncture, herbal medicines, and Tai Chi. The focus is on balancing the body's energy (Qi) to maintain health.
3. **Reiki (Japan)**: A form of energy healing where practitioners use their hands to channel healing energy into the patient's body to promote physical and emotional well-being.
4. **Naturopathy (Global)**: This practice uses natural remedies like herbs, massage, and nutritional counseling to support the body's ability to heal itself.
5. **Thalassotherapy (France)**: Utilizes sea water, seaweed, and other marine elements in spa treatments to promote health and wellness.

In integrating these holistic practices into your life, you'll experience a richer, more balanced approach to health and wellness, honoring traditions from around the world while fostering your personal journey toward holistic living.

CHAPTER 11

Chapter 11: Holistic Health for Different Life Sta

Holistic health encompasses every stage of life, recognizing that individuals have unique physical, emotional, and spiritual needs as they age. From infancy to adulthood, holistic health practices can support and nurture people through their various life phases.

Infancy and Childhood: These stages are characterized by high energy, curiosity, and rapid growth. Infants and children are greatly influenced by their families and society. During these early years, a supportive and nurturing environment is crucial. Babies need their parents' concern, care, and encouragement to thrive. Attention to nutrition, sleep, immunization, and creating a sense of safety are essential for their development. Positive interactions, playful activities, and age-appropriate learning experiences help build a strong foundation.

Tips for Supporting Infants and Children:

1. **Balanced Diet:** Provide a variety of nutritious foods to support physical growth and cognitive development.

2. **Regular Sleep:** Establish sleep routines that ensure adequate rest. A well-rested child is more likely to be calm and focused.
3. **Emotional Support:** Offer love, patience, and encouragement. Positive reinforcement helps children build self-esteem and resilience.
4. **Play and Learning:** Encourage play and educational activities that stimulate the mind and body. Balance structured learning with free play to foster creativity.
5. **Routine Medical Care:** Keep up with regular health check-ups and immunizations to monitor and support overall health.

Adolescence: This period of life is marked by significant physical, emotional, and social changes. Adolescents often seek independence and develop their identities. Support from family, friends, and mentors is vital as they navigate these transitions. Encouraging healthy habits and providing guidance can help adolescents make informed choices.

Tips for Supporting Adolescents:

1. **Open Communication:** Keep lines of communication open. Listen without judgment and provide a safe space for them to express their thoughts and feelings.
2. **Healthy Lifestyle:** Promote balanced nutrition, regular physical activity, and good sleep hygiene. Encourage hobbies and activities that promote well-being.
3. **Emotional Intelligence:** Teach adolescents how to recognize and manage their emotions. Stress the importance of self-awareness and empathy.
4. **Positive Role Models:** Surround them with positive influences and role models who inspire and guide them.

5. **Goal Setting:** Help adolescents set realistic goals and support them in achieving their aspirations.

Adulthood: Adults face a variety of challenges and responsibilities, including career demands, family obligations, and social relationships. Maintaining holistic health during adulthood involves balancing these aspects while paying attention to physical, mental, and spiritual well-being.

Tips for Supporting Adults:

1. **Work-Life Balance:** Prioritize work-life balance to reduce stress and maintain overall health. Set boundaries and make time for relaxation and enjoyment.
2. **Continuing Education:** Encourage lifelong learning and skill development. This can bring a sense of fulfillment and personal growth.
3. **Self-Care:** Integrate self-care practices into daily routines. This includes exercise, healthy eating, mindfulness, and seeking medical care when needed.
4. **Social Connections:** Cultivate strong social connections and a support network. Positive relationships enhance emotional well-being.
5. **Spiritual Growth:** Pursue spiritual practices that align with personal beliefs. This can provide a sense of purpose and inner peace.

Elderly Age: The later years of life come with their own set of challenges and opportunities. Seniors may experience physical limitations and health issues, but this stage can also be a time of reflection, wisdom, and deepened spiritual connection. Supporting elderly individuals involves respecting their autonomy while providing the care they need.

Tips for Supporting the Elderly:

1. **Physical Health:** Encourage regular physical activity appropriate for their ability. Focus on mobility, strength, and balance exercises.
2. **Mental Stimulation:** Engage in activities that challenge the mind, such as puzzles, reading, and social interactions.
3. **Nutritional Support:** Ensure a balanced diet that meets their nutritional needs. Consider supplements if necessary.
4. **Social Engagement:** Foster social connections and community involvement to combat loneliness and isolation.
5. **Dignity and Respect:** Treat elderly individuals with dignity and respect. Value their life experiences and wisdom.

CHAPTER 12

Chapter 12: Holistic Approaches to Chronic Illness

Living with chronic illness, also known as persistent health problems, presents unique challenges. However, numerous holistic health and wellness strategies can assist in managing these conditions, targeting underlying health issues, and improving general well-being. The effectiveness of various approaches depends on the specific chronic disease and its severity.

Always remember that holistic approaches complement, not replace, the advice and support from licensed medical professionals. Their experience and insight are invaluable in managing health problems. Weighing the balance of power with various support options is essential.

Here are some holistic strategies for managing chronic illness:

1. **Nutrition and Diet**: A balanced diet rich in whole foods, fresh fruits, vegetables, lean proteins, and healthy fats can aid in managing chronic conditions. Anti-inflammatory foods like turmeric, leafy greens, and berries can help reduce symptoms related to inflammation.

2. **Exercise and Physical Activity**: Regular, gentle exercise can improve physical health and alleviate symptoms of chronic illness. Activities such as walking, swimming, and yoga can enhance flexibility, strength, and cardiovascular health.
3. **Mind-Body Practices**: Techniques such as mindfulness, meditation, and deep-breathing exercises can reduce stress and promote relaxation. These practices help manage pain and improve overall well-being.
4. **Herbal Remedies**: Herbal treatments like ginger, garlic, and aloe vera can support health. Always consult with a healthcare provider before starting any new herbal regimen to ensure it doesn't interfere with existing treatments.
5. **Acupuncture and Acupressure**: These traditional Chinese medicine practices can help manage pain and improve energy flow within the body. They offer a non-invasive way to address chronic symptoms.
6. **Massage Therapy**: Regular massage can alleviate muscle tension, improve circulation, and promote relaxation. Specialized techniques like lymphatic drainage massage can also be beneficial.
7. **Hydrotherapy**: Using water in various forms (baths, showers, compresses) can soothe pain and inflammation. Warm baths with Epsom salts can relax muscles and promote detoxification.
8. **Aromatherapy**: Essential oils like lavender, peppermint, and eucalyptus can help manage pain, reduce stress, and improve sleep. Diffusing these oils or applying them topically can provide therapeutic benefits.
9. **Chiropractic Care**: Chiropractic adjustments can help manage pain and improve mobility, particularly for those with chronic back pain or joint issues.

10. **Emotional Support and Counseling**: Chronic illness can take a toll on mental health, so seeking emotional support and counseling is crucial. Therapy, support groups, and talking to trusted friends or family can help.
11. **Energy Healing**: Practices like Reiki or healing touch can balance energy and promote relaxation, aiding overall healing processes.
12. **Lifestyle Modifications**: Making lifestyle changes such as quitting smoking, reducing alcohol consumption, and maintaining a healthy weight can positively impact chronic illness management.

Incorporating these holistic strategies into your daily life can significantly enhance your ability to manage chronic illness. Always maintain open communication with your healthcare providers and ensure that any new holistic practices complement your existing treatment plan.

CHAPTER 13

Chapter 13: Integrating Holistic Practices into Da

The essence of leading a holistic lifestyle lies in the philosophy of daily habits. Examining and deciding what daily habits should be is a powerful and essential exercise of identifying which aspects of holistic living are most important to you. Acknowledging daily practices and other aspects of holistic living can provide a comforting routine, bringing more meaning and mindfulness into your life.

Instead of getting bogged down by abstract terms, focus on a collection of practices that vividly remind you of the simple, natural essence of holistic living. This daily commitment fosters self-respect, empathy, and a connection with the earth and your subconscious.

Here are some holistic daily practices to integrate into your life:

1. **Morning Rituals:** Start your day with mindfulness. Dedicate time in the morning to practices like meditation, yoga, or gratitude journaling. These rituals set a positive tone for the day.
2. **Nourishing Meals:** Eat mindfully, choosing whole, organic foods that nourish your body. Pay attention to how you feel while eating, and appreciate the flavors and nutrients.

3. **Physical Movement:** Make physical activity a regular part of your daily routine. This could be a morning walk, a session of Tai Chi, or a dance break in your living room. Movement keeps your energy balanced and your body strong.
4. **Mindful Breathing:** Pause throughout the day to practice deep, mindful breathing. This can reduce stress and bring you back to the present moment.
5. **Nature Connection:** Spend time outdoors as much as possible. Whether it's gardening, hiking, or simply enjoying a quiet moment in a park, nature has a grounding and healing effect.
6. **Balanced Work and Rest:** Create a balance between work and rest. Take regular breaks during work hours, and ensure you have downtime to unwind and relax.
7. **Minimalist Living:** Simplify your environment and surroundings by decluttering and organizing. A minimalist space reduces stress and promotes clarity.
8. **Evening Reflection:** End your day with reflective practices. Write in a journal, meditate, or read something inspiring. Reflect on the day's events, and express gratitude for the positives.
9. **Self-Care Routine:** Incorporate self-care activities into your daily schedule. This could be a relaxing bath, reading your favorite book, or pursuing a hobby you love.
10. **Acts of Kindness:** Perform small acts of kindness each day. Whether it's a smile, a kind word, or a helping hand, these actions enhance your own well-being and positively impact others.

As you weave these practices into your daily routine, your holistic beliefs will grow stronger, setting the stage for an overflow of good health, inner happiness, and all-around affection. You are the caretaker of your life, and these habits will help you stay connected to the energy, fresh air, and light that define a holistic lifestyle.

CHAPTER 14

Chapter 14: Holistic Wellness and the Workplace By

Holistic wellness in the workplace means finding personal balance and maintaining it in a daily rhythm. It involves understanding and integrating your physical and emotional needs with your professional role, allowing yourself to evolve and change. It means growing in the spirit of human progress and respecting your unique workplace growth pattern. Creating a balance between personal and professional life is crucial, but it can be challenging due to the myriad of factors at play. This balance can be compromised when we become overwhelmed at work or focus solely on professional commitments, often neglecting our own well-being.

Strategies for Achieving Workplace Wellness:

1. **Set Boundaries:** Establish clear boundaries between work and personal life. Define specific work hours and stick to them as much as possible, especially when working remotely.
2. **Prioritize Self-Care:** Make time for self-care activities during the day. Short breaks for mindfulness, stretching, or a walk can rejuvenate your mind and body.

3. **Create a Supportive Work Environment:** Foster positive relationships with colleagues and supervisors. A supportive work environment can alleviate stress and enhance job satisfaction.
4. **Flexible Working Arrangements:** Whenever possible, advocate for flexible working arrangements that accommodate personal needs without compromising professional responsibilities.
5. **Efficient Time Management:** Organize tasks effectively by prioritizing and scheduling your workload. Use tools like to-do lists, planners, or digital apps to stay on track.
6. **Health and Wellness Programs:** Engage in wellness programs offered by your organization. These can include fitness classes, mental health resources, and healthy eating initiatives.
7. **Open Communication:** Maintain open lines of communication with your employer and peers. Discuss any challenges you face and seek support when necessary.
8. **Work-Life Integration:** Strive for integration rather than balance by blending work responsibilities with personal life demands in a way that suits your lifestyle.
9. **Mental Health Support:** Utilize mental health resources if needed. Therapy, counseling, or employee assistance programs (EAPs) can provide valuable support.
10. **Physical Workspace:** Ensure your physical workspace is comfortable and conducive to productivity. Ergonomic furniture, proper lighting, and minimal distractions can make a significant difference.

Challenges During the Pandemic:

Creating balance between personal and professional life has become particularly difficult during the ongoing pandemic. Many people are working remotely while also caring for children or assisting with online education. Consistent internet access is paramount, yet often interrupted, leading to increased stress during work hours.

For those beginning to return to physical workplaces, concurrent demands for child care and financial considerations can add stress about re-establishing their former working life. Work-related stress is particularly challenging for parents who may experience it while their children are home and needing immediate attention. This stress can lead to negative energy, misunderstandings, and communication disruptions that impact both work and home environments.

Tips for Managing Pandemic-Related Work Stress:

1. **Routine and Structure:** Maintain a daily routine to provide stability for yourself and your family. Clearly separate work hours from personal time.
2. **Seek Support:** Reach out to family, friends, and colleagues for support. Sharing your experiences and coping strategies can lighten the load.
3. **Digital Detox:** Occasionally disconnect from digital devices to reduce screen fatigue and re-energize.
4. **Adaptability:** Embrace change and remain flexible. Adaptability can help you navigate new challenges more effectively.
5. **Focus on the Positive:** Shift your focus to the positive aspects of remote work, such as reduced commute times and increased family time.

By integrating these practices into your daily work life, you can create a healthier, more balanced approach to professional and personal wellness. Holistic wellness is about fostering resilience and adapting to new challenges while maintaining your well-being.

CHAPTER 15

Chapter 15: Holistic Wellness for Families and Chi

Sustainable well-being depends on a multitude of intersecting factors that influence every aspect of our lives. These factors play a crucial role in children's lives too, although integrating holistic wellness into their routines can be challenging with competing pressures and fast-paced lifestyles. In the United States, a staggering 60% of children's daily calories come from nutrient-depleting snack foods, often laden with toxins and pesticides. A 2004 EPA report detected 303 chemicals in the umbilical cord blood of babies born in the U.S.

As they grow, children are subjected to ever-increasing levels of stress—from academic performance pressure to the constant stimuli from TV, the Internet, and video games. Society's relentless push for academic excellence, coupled with rising mental health issues, makes it imperative to address wellness in all areas of a child's life: physical, mental, emotional, and spiritual.

Physical Wellness:

1. **Nutritious Diet**: Prioritize whole, organic foods free from harmful chemicals. Aim for balanced meals that include fruits, vegetables, lean proteins, and healthy fats. Educate children about the importance of nutrition.
2. **Exercise**: Encourage regular physical activity to promote strength, endurance, and flexibility. Activities like sports, outdoor play, and dance can make exercise fun.
3. **Rest**: Ensure children get adequate sleep. Establish a consistent bedtime routine to help them wind down and get quality rest.
4. **Clean Environment**: Minimize exposure to toxins by choosing natural cleaning products and reducing plastic use. Regularly clean living spaces to create a healthy home environment.

Mental Wellness:

1. **Life of Learning**: Foster a love for learning beyond academic pressure. Encourage curiosity through books, hands-on experiences, and creative pursuits. Emphasize the joy of discovery rather than academic performance.
2. **Stress Management**: Teach children stress-reduction techniques such as mindfulness, deep breathing, and time management. Support them in balancing schoolwork with relaxation and play.
3. **Technology Moderation**: Limit screen time and encourage tech-free activities. Promote face-to-face interactions and outdoor play to provide a break from digital stimuli.

Emotional Wellness:

1. **Emotional Support**: Offer consistent love, care, and encouragement. Create a safe space for children to express their emotions and listen without judgment.
2. **Positive Relationships**: Foster healthy relationships with family, friends, and peers. Teach empathy, kindness, and effective communication.
3. **Behavioral Guidance**: Use positive reinforcement to guide behavior. Set clear boundaries and consequences while maintaining open communication.

Spiritual Wellness:

1. **Inner Connection**: Encourage practices that help children connect with their inner selves, such as mindfulness meditation or quiet reflection.
2. **Values and Beliefs**: Share and model the family's values and beliefs. Provide opportunities for children to explore their spiritual interests and develop a sense of purpose.
3. **Nature and Reflection**: Spend time in nature and encourage children to appreciate the beauty and tranquility of the natural world. Reflecting on nature's wonders can deepen their spiritual awareness.

By weaving these holistic practices into the fabric of daily life, families can create a nurturing environment that supports children's overall well-being. The goal is not to isolate any one aspect but to address wellness comprehensively, ensuring children grow up healthy, balanced, and resilient.

CHAPTER 16

Chapter 16: Holistic Health and Aging Gracefully B

For those of us who are on this Earth for more than a few decades, aging is one of life's biggest challenges. Chronic diseases, lifestyle changes, and an increased need for self-care and exercise are part of that journey. Embracing holistic health provides a solid foundation to approach aging with joy and vitality. It's a conscious choice to age joyfully and healthily or to let the years weigh us down. To age gracefully means asking: What does my body, mind, and soul need to thrive?

Embrace Holistic Health Practices:

1. **Nutritional Excellence:** Focus on a nutrient-rich diet that supports overall health. Incorporate plenty of fruits, vegetables, whole grains, lean proteins, and healthy fats. Consider superfoods such as berries, nuts, and leafy greens to boost your nutrient intake.
2. **Regular Exercise:** Engage in physical activities that enhance flexibility, strength, and cardiovascular health. Brisk walking,

yoga, swimming, and resistance training can keep your body strong and agile.

3. **Mental Wellness:** Prioritize mental health by staying mentally active. Puzzles, reading, learning new skills, and engaging in social activities can keep your mind sharp. Practicing mindfulness and meditation helps manage stress and promotes inner peace.
4. **Emotional Balance:** Foster emotional well-being by nurturing positive relationships and seeking support when needed. Engaging in meaningful activities and maintaining a sense of purpose can enhance emotional stability.
5. **Spiritual Growth:** Cultivate a deep connection with your spiritual self. Engage in practices that resonate with you, such as prayer, meditation, or spending time in nature. Spiritual growth can provide a sense of fulfillment and tranquility.
6. **Holistic Healthcare:** Embrace holistic healthcare approaches that support physical, mental, and emotional balance. Regular check-ups, alternative therapies, and preventive measures can promote overall wellness.
7. **Regenerative Sleep:** Ensure you get adequate, restful sleep. Create a bedtime routine that promotes relaxation and maintain a sleep-friendly environment. Good sleep is crucial for rejuvenation and energy.
8. **Personal Growth:** Continue to pursue personal growth and self-discovery. Set goals, explore new interests, and challenge yourself to step out of your comfort zone. Personal growth contributes to a rich and fulfilling life.
9. **Reflection and Healing:** Work through past experiences and emotions to find healing and closure. Reflect on your life journey and embrace the lessons learned. This process can lead to emotional liberation and inner harmony.

Holistic health is not merely the absence of illness but the presence of maximum physical, mental, and emotional well-being. It's a way of life that integrates healthy eating, personal growth, meaningful relationships, honest emotional expression, regular physical activity, mental relaxation, regenerative sleep, and healing from past experiences.

As we age gracefully, we acknowledge the inevitable changes while celebrating the wisdom and growth that come with each passing year. Embracing holistic health ensures that our later years are vibrant, fulfilling, and filled with joy.

CHAPTER 17

Chapter 17: The Science Behind Holistic Healing By

Holistic belief posits that illness and suffering stem from mental, emotional, and spiritual imbalances, as well as maladaptation to the environment. Thus, healing shifts its focus from merely fighting disease to fostering overall wellness. The prevention of illness is viewed as the most effective pathway to wellness. Physical injury, for example, can be influenced by an individual's state of mind and emotional conditions. Many studies have demonstrated connections between heart disease and hostility, emotional stress and the immune system, belief and the immune system, and prolonged emotional stress with the onset of diseases like cancer due to immune suppression.

Research shows that prolonged conflict can tax the immune system and potentially induce conditions such as chronic fatigue syndrome. The medical establishment gradually acknowledges the profound interplay between mind, body, and spirit.

Scientific Insights into Holistic Healing:

1. **Mind-Body Connection:** The concept that the mind influences physical health is well-documented. Stress, depression, and anxiety can lead to physiological changes, affecting the immune system, cardiovascular health, and more. Techniques like mindfulness and meditation help manage stress and prevent related diseases.
2. **Role of Emotions:** Emotional health significantly impacts physical health. Positive emotions like joy, gratitude, and love can boost immune function, while negative emotions like anger and sadness can suppress it. Cultivating emotional well-being through therapy, social interactions, and hobbies can enhance overall health.
3. **Spiritual Beliefs:** Spiritual practices often contribute to holistic healing. Prayer, meditation, and spiritual rituals can provide comfort, reduce pain, and promote a sense of peace. These practices are linked to improved mental and physical health outcomes.
4. **Environmental Influence:** The environment plays a crucial role in holistic health. Factors such as air quality, access to green spaces, and exposure to pollutants can impact health. Creating a balanced environment by reducing exposure to toxins and fostering a connection with nature can support well-being.

Holistic Healing Practices:

1. **Integrative Medicine:** Combining conventional medical treatments with holistic practices can provide comprehensive care. This approach considers the whole person, addressing physical, emotional, and spiritual aspects.

2. **Herbal Medicine:** Herbs like turmeric, ginger, and echinacea have been used for centuries to promote healing. Scientific research supports their efficacy in reducing inflammation, boosting immunity, and more.
3. **Energy Healing:** Practices like Reiki and acupuncture aim to balance the body's energy flow. These techniques are believed to restore harmony and support physical and emotional healing.
4. **Nutrition:** A balanced diet rich in nutrients supports the body's natural healing processes. Anti-inflammatory foods, antioxidants, and adequate hydration play key roles in maintaining health.
5. **Exercise:** Regular physical activity promotes cardiovascular health, strengthens muscles, and enhances mental well-being. Yoga, tai chi, and other movement practices also support emotional and spiritual balance.

Future Perspectives in Holistic Healing:

In today's world, we no longer limit ourselves to alleviating suffering or treating illness. We strive to create mental, emotional, and environmental balance to help prevent disease. By identifying triggers and chemicals that influence the soul and spirit, we can help individuals achieve personal wellness through environmental balance.

As evolved beings on this planet, we now have the ability to create and maintain personal wellness rather than waiting for disease to manifest. This represents one of the greatest gifts of holistic healing—the belief that healing is not just about curing disease and suffering but about achieving comprehensive well-being and universal health. Healing the soul can lead to healing the body, emphasizing the interconnectedness of our existence.

CHAPTER 18

Chapter 18: Holistic Therapies and Alternative Med

Holistic therapies and alternative medicine offer natural, gentle ways to heal the body and mind, enhance beauty, and manage stress. These approaches often provide a relaxing alternative to conventional treatments, making them appealing to many seeking balance and well-being.

Aromatherapy uses natural ingredients like essential oils to promote healing and relaxation. The therapeutic properties of these oils can offer relief from stress, support the immune system, and enhance overall wellness. With its soothing effects, aromatherapy is perfect for people looking to unwind and restore balance.

Nutritional Therapy is a drug-free approach to boosting the immune system. It emphasizes detoxification, supported by a healthy diet and nutritional supplements. This therapy involves a comprehensive, individualized diet plan and careful supplementation to provide the body with essential nutrients, aiding in the detoxification process.

In holistic healing, patients are seen as whole beings, not just a collection of symptoms. Treatment encompasses mental and physical well-being, offering a relaxed atmosphere, wholesome food, massages, yoga, and acupuncture. Addressing stress and everyday pressures is central to holistic care, as unmanaged stress can weaken the body's defenses and lead to illness.

Holistic Therapies:

1. **Acupuncture:** This traditional Chinese medicine practice involves inserting thin needles into specific points on the body to balance energy flow and alleviate pain. It can support the treatment of various ailments, including chronic pain, anxiety, and digestive issues.
2. **Massage Therapy:** Regular massages can reduce muscle tension, improve circulation, and promote relaxation. Techniques like Swedish, deep tissue, and lymphatic drainage can be tailored to individual needs.
3. **Reiki:** A form of energy healing, Reiki involves a practitioner placing their hands on or near the patient's body to channel healing energy. It aims to restore balance and promote physical and emotional well-being.
4. **Homeopathy:** This system of medicine uses highly diluted substances to stimulate the body's natural healing processes. It is based on the principle of "like cures like," where a substance that causes symptoms in a healthy person can treat similar symptoms in a sick person.
5. **Herbal Medicine:** The use of plant-based remedies can support various health conditions. Herbs like echinacea, ginseng, and chamomile are known for their healing properties.
6. **Chiropractic Care:** Focused on diagnosing and treating mechanical disorders of the musculoskeletal system, particularly the spine, chiropractic care can help alleviate back pain, improve joint function, and enhance overall health.

Alternative Medicine:

1. **Ayurveda:** This ancient Indian system of medicine emphasizes balance and harmony in the body through diet, herbal treatments, and yogic practices. Ayurvedic principles focus on maintaining health and preventing illness by balancing the body's energies.
2. **Traditional Chinese Medicine (TCM):** TCM includes acupuncture, herbal medicine, and practices like Tai Chi and Qigong. It seeks to balance the body's energy (Qi) and promote overall health.
3. **Naturopathy:** Naturopathic medicine combines modern scientific knowledge with traditional practices. It emphasizes prevention, treatment, and optimal health through natural therapies, including nutrition, lifestyle counseling, and botanical medicine.

Access to Holistic Care:

Access to holistic and alternative care can vary widely. Those willing to invest in these therapies often have more choices, while many who could benefit most lack access. To bridge this gap, we must provide resources and information to make these practices more accessible.

Here's a list of valuable resources:

- **Books and Authors:** Renowned books and authors on holistic health (e.g., "The Complete Book of Essential Oils and Aromatherapy" by Valerie Ann Worwood).
- **Practitioners and Organizations:** Directories of certified holistic practitioners and reputable organizations.

- **Websites and Articles:** Online platforms offering detailed information on various holistic therapies and alternative medicine practices.
- **Workshops and Seminars:** Opportunities to learn more about holistic health practices through interactive sessions and expert talks.

By empowering individuals with knowledge and resources, we can help them make informed decisions and find the right holistic support. Living a balanced life is within reach for everyone, and holistic health practices can pave the way to wellness and harmony.

CHAPTER 19

Chapter 19: Holistic Living and Traditional Medici

The concepts of holistic living, holistic healing, and holistic health are deeply rooted in traditional medicine and the fundamental principles guiding it. These principles are also well-represented in contemporary health care models and practices. The renowned "Father of Medicine," Hippocrates, an ancient Greek physician who significantly impacted the course of medicine, endorsed holistic thinking and treatment over 2,400 years ago. He advised the ancient Greeks to consider the body, mind, and spirit as one cohesive entity in the healing process.

Hippocrates taught, as Holistic Medicine continues to teach today, that the whole person—the body, mind, and spirit—must be considered and treated. Illness is not merely about "broken" body parts but the balance or imbalance within the body, mind, feelings, and spirit. This interconnectedness is a foundational principle of Traditional Medicine, deeply rooted in Holistic Practice, and is also reflected in modern health care models.

Traditional Medicine Practices:

1. **Ayurveda (India):** This ancient system of medicine focuses on balance and harmony within the body through diet, herbal treatments, and yogic practices. Ayurvedic principles emphasize the prevention of illness and the maintenance of health by addressing the body's energies.
2. **Traditional Chinese Medicine (China):** TCM includes practices like acupuncture, herbal medicine, Tai Chi, and Qigong. It seeks to balance the body's Qi (energy) to maintain health and treat ailments.
3. **Native American Medicine (North America):** This practice involves the use of herbs, spirituality, and rituals to maintain balance and harmony within the body and with the environment.
4. **Unani Medicine (Persia):** Based on the teachings of Hippocrates, Galen, and Islamic scholars, Unani medicine emphasizes balance in the body's humors and the prevention of disease through lifestyle and diet.

Holistic Integration with Modern Health Care:

Modern health care models, such as the Comprehensive Health Model, emphasize the integration of holistic principles with contemporary medical practices. This approach considers the whole person and addresses multiple dimensions of health, including physical, mental, emotional, and spiritual well-being.

Principles of Holistic and Traditional Medicine:

1. **Whole-Person Care:** Both holistic and traditional medicine emphasize the importance of treating the whole person—addressing physical, mental, and spiritual aspects—to promote overall health and well-being.

2. **Balance and Harmony:** A key principle is maintaining balance and harmony within the body and with the environment. This principle guides both traditional practices like Ayurveda and TCM and modern holistic approaches.
3. **Prevention and Wellness:** Prevention is a core tenet, with an emphasis on maintaining health and preventing illness through lifestyle, diet, and natural remedies.
4. **Personalized Treatment:** Both approaches recognize that each individual is unique, and treatments should be personalized to meet their specific needs.
5. **Integration of Natural Remedies:** The use of natural remedies, such as herbs, dietary changes, and physical practices like yoga and Tai Chi, is common in both traditional and holistic medicine.

Modern Applications of Traditional Holistic Principles:

1. **Functional Medicine:** This modern medical practice adopts holistic principles by focusing on identifying and addressing the root causes of disease. It integrates traditional medical practices with contemporary clinical practices to provide personalized care.
2. **Integrative Medicine:** Combining traditional and modern medical practices, integrative medicine incorporates holistic principles to treat the whole person. It emphasizes the use of natural remedies, lifestyle changes, and mind-body practices alongside conventional treatments.
3. **Preventive Medicine:** This approach prioritizes prevention and wellness, aligning with holistic principles. Preventive medicine focuses on maintaining health, preventing illness,

and promoting overall well-being through lifestyle modifications and natural remedies.

Hippocrates' teachings, emphasizing the interconnectedness of the body, mind, and spirit, continue to influence holistic health practices today. By integrating these timeless principles with modern health care, we can create a comprehensive approach to health and wellness that honors the legacy of traditional medicine while embracing the innovations of contemporary practice.

CHAPTER 20

Chapter 20: Holistic Health and Preventive Care By

Maintaining health and wellness requires effort, persistence, and a self-motivated attitude. To avoid illness and enjoy a peaceful life filled with strength and vitality, it's important to follow some key guidelines. This "prescription" for health includes plenty of fresh air, clean water, and a nutritious diet filled with natural ingredients. Moderation, elimination habits, and exercise are crucial components of preventive care. But there's more to it than just the physical aspects—love, self-love, and vitality play essential roles too.

Sitting comfortably and truly listening to your body is a necessary skill for sensing pain, stiffness, strain, or fatigue. Engage in gentle movements, breathing exercises, and stretching daily. Aim to find time for fitness 4 to 5 times per week. Regular exercise and healthy eating habits improve the functioning of both the body and the mind. Spending time outside in nature lifts your spirit and renews your energy.

Building a Holistic Preventive Care Routine:

1. **Quality Nutrition:** Focus on consuming whole, organic foods that nourish your body. Include a variety of fruits, vegetables, lean proteins, and healthy fats in your diet.
2. **Regular Exercise:** Incorporate different forms of physical activity into your routine. Gentle stretching, yoga, walking, and strength training contribute to overall well-being.
3. **Adequate Hydration:** Drink plenty of clean water throughout the day to keep your body hydrated and functioning optimally.
4. **Breathing Techniques:** Practice deep breathing exercises to reduce stress and enhance mental clarity. Techniques like diaphragmatic breathing can promote relaxation.
5. **Spiritual Connection:** Spend time in nature and engage in activities that connect you to your spiritual self. Whether it's meditation, prayer, or quiet reflection, nurturing your spirit is essential.
6. **Social Support:** Let others support you in achieving your goals. Join groups, workout with a friend, or enjoy recreational activities with loved ones.
7. **Rest and Relaxation:** Balance activity with quiet time alone. Give yourself permission to rest and recharge away from the demands of daily life.
8. **Positive Self-Image:** Maintain a constructive self-image by focusing on your strengths and accomplishments. Embrace self-love and celebrate your uniqueness.
9. **Mindfulness:** Savor each moment and appreciate the little things in life. Practice mindfulness to stay present and grounded.
10. **Regular Health Checks:** Schedule routine physical checkups and screenings, even when you feel well. Preventive medical care helps catch potential issues early.

Incorporating these practices into your daily life can lead to a harmonious balance of the mind, body, and spirit. Engaging in activities you enjoy keeps you active and helps manage feelings of sadness and stress. A joyous and fulfilling life is within reach when you summon romance, wonder, delight, and magic into your heart.

Your life is filled with unique, unrepeatable moments that deserve your attention and presence. Take the time to reflect on who you want to become and what will make you genuinely happy in the long run. Your long-term goals and beliefs are crucial in shaping your health and well-being.

No one understands your needs and aspirations better than you do. While healthcare professionals offer valuable advice and support, you are the architect of your health journey. Preventive care is not just about avoiding illness but about creating a life brimming with health, happiness, and vitality.

CHAPTER 21

Chapter 21: Holistic Wellness Retreats and Centers

One of the most renowned holistic wellness retreats in the world is the Sanoviv Medical Institute, a tranquil haven overlooking the sea in Baja, Mexico. Offering a comprehensive five-week mind-body-heart cleanse, known as the Ultimate Wellness Plan, Sanoviv is unique in the world of holistic wellness retreats. At peak times, Sanoviv accommodates up to 40 guests, supported by ten skilled practitioners and a robust team of 200 for exceptional care and service.

The Sanoviv Experience:

Upon arrival at Sanoviv, each guest is assigned a personal Wellness Coordinator to guide them through their individualized programs. This bespoke plan includes:

- **Medical Assessments**: Comprehensive evaluations to understand each guest's health status.
- **Individual Lab Work**: Personalized testing to identify specific health needs.

- **Nutritional Consultations**: Detailed discussions with a doctor to develop a tailored diet plan.
- **Healing Modalities**: Access to over 40 different therapies and treatments.
- **Educational Classes**: Informative sessions on various aspects of holistic health.
- **Chef Demonstrations**: Interactive cooking classes showcasing nutritious organic cuisine.
- **Spa Treatments**: Luxurious therapies to promote relaxation and rejuvenation.
- **Organic Cuisine**: Freshly prepared meals tailored to meet individual dietary requirements.
- **Life Coaching**: Personal development sessions to set and achieve life goals.
- **Personal Training**: Customized fitness plans to enhance physical health.
- **Journaling**: Guided exercises to encourage reflection and mindfulness.

After the five-week Ultimate Wellness Plan, guests receive continued support from Sanoviv's aftercare practitioners to ensure they remain healthy and follow the program at home. This holistic approach ensures lasting benefits for the mind, body, and spirit.

Other Holistic Wellness Retreats:

While Sanoviv is exceptional, numerous other retreats around the world offer unique holistic wellness experiences:

1. **The Raj (Fairfield, Iowa, USA)**: This Ayurvedic retreat provides personalized wellness programs based on ancient healing traditions. Their offerings include Panchakarma detox, meditation, yoga, and nutritional counseling.

2. **Ananda in the Himalayas (Uttarakhand, India)**: Known for its luxurious spa treatments and stunning location, this retreat emphasizes Ayurvedic and Western wellness techniques. Guests can enjoy yoga, meditation, and personalized health consultations.
3. **Kamalaya (Koh Samui, Thailand)**: This award-winning wellness sanctuary focuses on holistic healing and lifestyle enhancement. Programs include detox, stress management, and emotional balance, supported by traditional therapies and modern medical practices.
4. **SHA Wellness Clinic (Alicante, Spain)**: Combining Eastern and Western treatments, SHA offers a range of wellness programs, including detox, weight loss, and anti-aging. Their integrative approach ensures a comprehensive healing experience.

Benefits of Holistic Wellness Retreats:

Holistic wellness retreats provide a serene environment away from daily stresses, allowing individuals to focus on improving their well-being. These retreats offer:

- **Customized Care**: Personalized plans tailored to individual health needs.
- **Comprehensive Treatments**: A blend of traditional and modern therapies addressing physical, mental, and spiritual health.
- **Expert Guidance**: Access to skilled practitioners and wellness experts.
- **Healthy Environment**: Stress-free settings that promote relaxation and healing.

- **Long-term Benefits**: Continued support and guidance to maintain wellness after returning home.

Sanoviv Medical Institute, along with these other esteemed retreats, serve as sanctuaries for those seeking to recalibrate and restore their health. By embracing the holistic approach, guests can return with renewed energy, clarity, and a balanced perspective on life.

CHAPTER 22

Chapter 22: Holistic Living and Mindfulness Practi

Holistic living can be a journey of both simplicity and complexity. While some aspects may become easier, others can challenge us in beautiful ways. Simplicity and openness keep life engaging, as each of us must find our own answers and paths.

Mindfulness practices are essential tools in the search for tranquility, increased awareness, and balance in a stressful world. Spending time in nature, practicing meditation, embracing mindfulness, and cultivating qualities like loving-kindness and compassion all contribute to achieving a state of enlightenment. These practices don't require commitment to any religious or philosophical beliefs, allowing anyone to integrate them into their lives.

Key Mindfulness Practices for Holistic Living:

1. **Nature Connection:** Spending time in natural surroundings can ground your energy and provide a sense of peace. Whether through hiking, gardening, or simply sitting in a park, nature offers a respite from daily stress.

2. **Meditation:** Regular meditation practice helps quiet the mind and connect with your inner self. Techniques can include breath-focused meditation, guided imagery, or body scan meditations.
3. **Mindful Breathing:** Simple yet powerful, mindful breathing exercises can reduce stress and bring you into the present moment. Practice deep, mindful breaths throughout the day to refocus your mind.
4. **Loving-Kindness (Metta) Meditation:** This practice involves sending love and goodwill to yourself and others. It can help cultivate compassion and transform negative emotions into positive ones.
5. **Gratitude Journaling:** Writing down what you are grateful for each day can shift your mindset and help you appreciate the positives in your life.
6. **Mindful Movement:** Activities like yoga, Tai Chi, or even mindful walking integrate physical movement with mindfulness, promoting both physical and mental wellness.

As we practice mindfulness, we can open the door to more complex behaviors, raising our awareness of our interconnectedness with all beings. Mindfulness teachings and practices, dating back to the time of the Buddha, have become mainstream in the modern world. They offer practical ways to increase awareness, gently guide our thoughts and actions without judgment, and foster a sense of inner peace.

These timeless teachings don't demand adherence to any dogma; instead, they resonate with us on a personal level. If we hope to seek tranquility, compassion, and alignment, we can adapt these practices to our lives, ceasing to fuel the unrest that disrupts our well-being.

Integrating Mindfulness into Daily Life:

1. **Start Small:** Begin with a few minutes of mindfulness or meditation each day, gradually increasing the duration as you become more comfortable.
2. **Consistent Practice:** Like any skill, mindfulness requires consistency. Make it a regular part of your routine to see long-term benefits.
3. **Non-Judgmental Awareness:** Practice observing your thoughts and feelings without judgment. Accept them as they are and let them pass without attachment.
4. **Mindful Eating:** Pay attention to the flavors, textures, and sensations of your food. Eating mindfully can enhance your appreciation of meals and improve digestion.
5. **Mindful Listening:** When conversing with others, practice active listening. Focus on their words without planning your response, creating deeper connections.

By integrating these mindful practices into your daily life, you can enhance your holistic living journey, finding greater peace, balance, and awareness in every moment.

CHAPTER 23

Chapter 23: Holistic Approaches to Pain Management

Pain can dominate life, affecting our activities, relationships, and decision-making. Millions suffer from chronic pain, making it a primary reason for doctor visits. Conventional treatments like medications and surgery can be invasive, expensive, and may not always provide relief. Excessive use of pain medications can also lead to significant health problems. Alternative, holistic pain management approaches emphasize healing pain at its source and addressing underlying imbalances, rather than just relieving symptoms. Many are non-invasive and provide effective strategies that align with the mind-body interaction.

Holistic Pain Relief Strategies:

1. **Mind-Body Techniques:** Practices like meditation, mindfulness, and biofeedback can help manage pain by promoting relaxation and altering the perception of pain. These techniques train the brain to respond differently to pain signals.
2. **Acupuncture:** This ancient Chinese medicine practice involves inserting thin needles into specific points on the body

to balance energy flow and alleviate pain. It has been effective in treating various pain conditions such as migraines and chronic pain.

3. **Herbal Remedies:** Herbs like turmeric, ginger, and willow bark have natural anti-inflammatory properties that can help reduce pain. Always consult with a healthcare provider before starting any herbal regimen.
4. **Physical Therapy:** Regular physical therapy sessions can help improve mobility, strengthen muscles, and reduce pain. Physical therapists use techniques such as massage, stretching, and exercise to address pain at its source.
5. **Chiropractic Care:** Chiropractic adjustments can help alleviate pain by correcting misalignments in the spine and improving joint function. This approach is particularly effective for back and neck pain.
6. **Nutritional Therapy:** A balanced diet rich in essential nutrients can support the body's natural healing processes. Reducing inflammatory foods and increasing intake of anti-inflammatory foods can help manage pain.
7. **Yoga and Tai Chi:** These gentle exercises promote flexibility, balance, and relaxation. They can help reduce pain by improving circulation and reducing stress.
8. **Aromatherapy:** Essential oils like lavender, peppermint, and eucalyptus can help manage pain and promote relaxation. Diffusing these oils or applying them topically can provide therapeutic benefits.
9. **Massage Therapy:** Regular massages can reduce muscle tension, improve circulation, and promote relaxation. Techniques like Swedish and deep tissue massage can be tailored to individual needs.

10. **Energy Healing:** Practices like Reiki and healing touch aim to balance the body's energy flow, promote relaxation, and reduce pain.

Restoring Harmony and Balance:

1. **Awareness and Understanding:** The first step in holistic pain management is increasing awareness and understanding of the different sources of pain and the mind-body interaction. Pain can signal physical imbalances and guide us toward addressing mental, emotional, or spiritual issues.
2. **Addressing Sources of Pain:** Identifying and addressing the root causes of pain is crucial. This may involve lifestyle changes, stress management, and adopting healthier habits.
3. **Nutrition and Detoxification:** Painful conditions such as migraines, sinus issues, urinary and digestive disorders can often be alleviated with dietary changes, body detoxification, and increased intake of essential nutrients.
4. **Perspective and Symbolism:** Our perspective shapes pain because it works according to symbolic rules. Viewing pain as a guide, rather than a dictator, requires conscious awareness of our actions and their symbolic meanings.

Creating a Holistic Pain Management Plan:

1. **Consult a Holistic Practitioner:** Seek guidance from a holistic healthcare provider who can help develop a personalized pain management plan.
2. **Incorporate Multiple Strategies:** Use a combination of techniques like mindfulness, acupuncture, nutritional therapy, and physical therapy for a comprehensive approach.

3. **Monitor Progress:** Keep track of pain levels, triggers, and the effectiveness of different strategies. Adjust your plan as needed to ensure optimal results.
4. **Stay Consistent:** Holistic pain management requires consistency and commitment. Regular practice of these techniques can lead to lasting relief and improved quality of life.

By integrating these holistic strategies into daily life, you can restore harmony, balance, and tempo, ultimately reducing pain and enhancing overall well-being. Embrace the journey toward a pain-free, balanced life with holistic practices guiding the way.

CHAPTER 24

Chapter 24: Holistic Beauty and Skincare By Nolan

To elevate our holistic living philosophies, it's essential to look beyond what we put into our bodies and focus on what we put onto our bodies. While holistic living starts from the inside out, our skin, the largest organ of the body, plays a crucial role in our overall health, well-being, and appearance. Nourishing and maintaining our skin, hair, and nails with healthy, natural, non-toxic skincare products is essential for a balanced lifestyle. Believe it or not, it takes just twenty seconds for chemicals in personal skincare products to penetrate into our bloodstream, which can sometimes be more detrimental to our health than smoking.

Principles of Holistic Skincare:

1. **Natural Ingredients:** Choose skincare products made from natural, non-toxic ingredients. Look for items free of harmful chemicals like parabens, sulfates, and synthetic fragrances. Ingredients like aloe vera, coconut oil, and chamomile are gentle and beneficial.

2. **Organic Products:** Opt for organic skincare products that are free from pesticides and GMOs. Organic products ensure that you are not applying harmful chemicals to your skin.
3. **Eco-Friendly Choices:** Select products with environmentally friendly packaging and sustainable practices. Eco-friendly products help reduce your carbon footprint and protect the planet.
4. **Cruelty-Free Options:** Choose cruelty-free products that are not tested on animals. Ethical beauty practices contribute to a more compassionate world. Look for certifications like Leaping Bunny or PETA-approved.
5. **Fair Trade:** Support fair trade products that ensure fair wages and working conditions for producers. Fair trade practices promote ethical consumerism and social responsibility.

Holistic Skincare Routine:

1. **Cleanse:** Use a gentle, natural cleanser to remove impurities without stripping the skin of its natural oils. Cleansing helps maintain clear, healthy skin.
2. **Exfoliate:** Regular exfoliation removes dead skin cells and promotes cell turnover. Use natural exfoliants like sugar, oatmeal, or rice powder a couple of times a week.
3. **Tone:** Apply a natural toner to balance the skin's pH and tighten pores. Ingredients like witch hazel, rose water, or apple cider vinegar are effective options.
4. **Moisturize:** Hydrate your skin with a natural moisturizer that suits your skin type. Ingredients such as shea butter, jojoba oil, and hyaluronic acid provide deep hydration.

5. **Protect:** Always use a natural sunscreen to protect your skin from harmful UV rays. Look for physical sunscreens with ingredients like zinc oxide or titanium dioxide.
6. **Nourish:** Use natural serums or face oils to nourish your skin. Ingredients like vitamin C, rosehip oil, and argan oil can enhance radiance and address specific skin concerns.

Holistic Beauty Tips:

1. **Stay Hydrated:** Drink plenty of water throughout the day to keep your skin hydrated from the inside out. Proper hydration supports overall health and skin vitality.
2. **Balanced Diet:** Eat a balanced diet rich in vitamins, minerals, and antioxidants. Foods like berries, leafy greens, nuts, and seeds promote healthy, glowing skin.
3. **Rest and Relaxation:** Ensure you get adequate restful sleep. Sleep is essential for skin regeneration and overall well-being.
4. **Stress Management:** Manage stress through mindfulness, meditation, or yoga. Reducing stress can prevent skin issues like acne and premature aging.
5. **Physical Activity:** Regular physical activity improves circulation, bringing essential nutrients to the skin. Exercise contributes to a healthy, radiant complexion.

Mindful Skincare Choices:

- **Research Ingredients:** Always check the ingredient list of skincare products. Educate yourself about harmful chemicals and avoid products that contain them.
- **Choose Sustainable Brands:** Support brands that prioritize sustainability, ethical practices, and transparency.

- **DIY Skincare:** Consider making your own skincare products using natural ingredients. DIY options allow you to control what you put on your skin and customize recipes to suit your needs.

The Inner Glow:

True beauty comes from a healthy and radiant inner glow. Holistic beauty starts from within, with the key ingredients for youthful and vibrant looks being a balanced lifestyle, nutritious diet, and positive mindset. Mindful and conscious choices ensure the highest possible standards and quality practices in beauty, cosmetic, and skincare products and treatments. By choosing simple, pure, natural, safe, non-toxic, eco-friendly, organic, cruelty-free, and fair trade products, you embrace a holistic approach that benefits both your well-being and the environment.

CHAPTER 25

Chapter 25: Holistic Fitness Trends and Practices

Holistic fitness is gaining popularity as more people seek mindful fitness and diet routines. The goal is to integrate fitness into daily life while enhancing self-care. Holistic fitness routines bridge various aspects of well-being, including meditation, yoga, strength training, diet, skincare, mindfulness, and lifestyle habits.

Key Holistic Fitness Trends:

1. **Yoga:** Yoga remains a cornerstone of holistic fitness, offering numerous benefits such as increased flexibility, strength, and mental clarity. Different types of yoga, like Vinyasa, Hatha, and Bikram, cater to various fitness levels and preferences.
2. **Barre:** This ballet-inspired workout combines elements of dance, Pilates, and yoga. It focuses on small, controlled movements to tone muscles and improve posture. Barre classes often include upbeat music to keep the energy high.
3. **POUND®:** This unique fitness trend combines cardio and strength training with drumming. Using lightly weighted

drumsticks called Ripstix®, participants engage in a full-body workout that burns calories and relieves stress.

4. **Tai Chi:** Particularly popular among Baby Boomers, Tai Chi is a gentle martial art that promotes balance, flexibility, and mental calmness. It involves slow, deliberate movements and deep breathing, making it accessible to people of all fitness levels.
5. **Yoga Therapy:** This specialized form of yoga focuses on the therapeutic aspects, addressing specific health issues and promoting overall well-being. It combines traditional yoga practices with modern medical knowledge.

Holistic Living Practices:

1. **Mindfulness Meditation:** Incorporating mindfulness meditation into your fitness routine enhances mental clarity and reduces stress. This practice encourages you to stay present and focused during your workouts.
2. **Strength Training:** Holistic fitness includes strength training exercises that build muscle, improve metabolism, and support overall health. Combining weights or resistance bands with bodyweight exercises can create a balanced routine.
3. **Diet and Nutrition:** A holistic approach to fitness emphasizes a healthy, balanced diet. Incorporating whole foods, staying hydrated, and avoiding processed foods can improve energy levels and overall well-being.
4. **Skincare:** Taking care of your skin is an integral part of holistic fitness. Using natural, non-toxic skincare products ensures that your skin remains healthy and radiant.

Summer's Holistic Fitness Trends:

1. **Holistic Business Chats:** Engaging in discussions about holistic living, fitness, and wellness with experts and enthusiasts. These chats offer valuable insights and inspiration to enhance your holistic lifestyle.
2. **Fermentation Fun:** Exploring the benefits of fermented foods like kimchi, sauerkraut, and kombucha. These probiotic-rich foods support digestive health and boost the immune system.
3. **Meditation Musings on Mindfulness and Eating:** Integrating mindful eating practices into your daily routine. This approach encourages you to savor each bite and recognize the body's hunger and fullness cues.
4. **Diet Bits and Bites:** Sharing tips and recipes for nutritious, balanced meals. Emphasizing the importance of a varied diet that includes plenty of fruits, vegetables, lean proteins, and healthy fats.

CHC Class in Holistic Fitness:

Completing a comprehensive holistic fitness class, like the CHC (Certified Holistic Coach) class, can provide you with deeper knowledge and practical skills. These classes cover various aspects of holistic health, including fitness, nutrition, mindfulness, and lifestyle choices.

By embracing holistic fitness trends and practices, you can create a balanced, healthy lifestyle that nurtures both body and mind. Incorporating these practices into your daily routine will help you achieve overall well-being and take on the world with renewed energy and confidence.

CHAPTER 26

Chapter 26: Holistic Health and Herbal Medicine By

In a truly holistic approach to health, it's essential to treat the body's imbalances by recognizing patterns of illness and using appropriate remedies. Herbal medicine is unique among healing traditions because it treats the individual as a living ecosystem. This approach uses plants whose signature manifestations resemble the patterns of illness they treat. For example, hawthorn berries, with their heart-like shape and their growth around the heart areas of different plants, are beneficial for the circulatory system.

Herbal medicine works on the principle that the body is an ecosystem made up of millions of other living ecosystems. Surprisingly, only 10% of the body's cells are human, and a mere 1% of the body's DNA is specifically human; the rest is bacterial, viral, or fungal in origin. This understanding of our existence as complex, interdependent ecosystems makes it easier to grasp the concept of plant spirits. Plants, essential to the ecosystem, become part of our bodies and help restore balance within our personal ecosystems and the larger ecosystem around us.

Principles of Herbal Medicine:

1. **Pattern Recognition:** Herbalists identify patterns of illness and choose plants with similar manifestations to treat those conditions. This approach aims to balance the body's internal ecosystem.
2. **Holistic Treatment:** Rather than focusing solely on symptoms, herbal medicine addresses the root causes of imbalances. It considers the physical, mental, emotional, and spiritual aspects of health.
3. **Natural Remedies:** Herbal medicine uses natural plant-based remedies to support healing. These remedies are often gentler on the body compared to synthetic medications.
4. **Individualized Care:** Treatment plans are tailored to the individual, recognizing that each person's ecosystem is unique. Herbalists take into account the individual's specific needs and constitution.

Common Herbs and Their Uses:

1. **Hawthorn:** Beneficial for the heart and circulatory system. It can help lower blood pressure, improve circulation, and strengthen the heart.
2. **Chamomile:** Known for its calming properties, chamomile can help with anxiety, insomnia, and digestive issues.
3. **Echinacea:** Boosts the immune system and helps fight off infections. It's commonly used to prevent colds and flu.
4. **Turmeric:** Contains anti-inflammatory properties and can help with conditions like arthritis and digestive disorders.
5. **Ginger:** Aids in digestion and relieves nausea. It's also known for its anti-inflammatory and antioxidant effects.
6. **Lavender:** Promotes relaxation and can help with stress, anxiety, and sleep disorders.

7. **Peppermint:** Useful for digestive issues, headaches, and respiratory problems. It has a cooling and soothing effect.
8. **Aloe Vera:** Known for its healing properties, aloe vera can soothe skin irritations, burns, and digestive issues.

Holistic Practices with Herbal Medicine:

1. **Herbal Teas:** Drinking herbal teas is a simple way to incorporate the benefits of herbs into your daily routine. Choose teas that target specific health needs or promote overall well-being.
2. **Tinctures and Extracts:** Concentrated herbal extracts can be taken in small amounts to address specific health issues. These are typically more potent than teas and can be customized to individual needs.
3. **Topical Applications:** Herbal balms, oils, and salves can be applied to the skin for localized relief of pain, inflammation, or skin conditions.
4. **Dietary Supplements:** Incorporating herbal supplements into your diet can provide additional support for various health concerns. Always consult with a healthcare provider before starting new supplements.
5. **Aromatherapy:** Using essential oils made from herbs can enhance mood, relieve stress, and support holistic health. Diffuse oils or apply them topically with a carrier oil.

Restoring Balance with Herbal Medicine:

Herbal medicine emphasizes the interconnectedness of all living things and the importance of maintaining balance within our personal ecosystems. By recognizing patterns of illness and using plants to restore harmony, herbalists help individuals achieve optimal health. This holistic approach aligns with the principles of holistic health, promoting a balanced and harmonious life.

CHAPTER 27

Chapter 27: Holistic Approaches to Detoxification

Detoxification, or internal cleansing, plays a vital role in promoting balance within the body. These holistic approaches help improve intestinal bacteria balance, enhance bowel function, correct imbalances such as mildew syndrome, and restore normal body chemistry and organ function.

Colon Irrigation: Also known as colon cleansing or colon hydrotherapy, this gentle and safe procedure involves washing the colon with warm water. The goal is to cleanse the few feet of the digestive tube that remain active after the digestion of useful nutrients. This approach can help clear up skin problems, promote weight loss, and improve overall bowel health.

Liver Detoxification: The liver, the body's master detoxifier and blood purifier, can be rejuvenated using painless, proven, and safe holistic methods such as castor oil packs and coffee enemas. These methods support liver function, aid in the elimination of toxins, and enhance overall well-being.

Holistic Detox Strategies:

1. **Whole Foods Diet:** Emphasize a diet rich in whole, organic foods that support the body's natural detox processes. Include plenty of fruits, vegetables, lean proteins, and whole grains to provide essential nutrients.
2. **Hydration:** Maintain proper hydration by drinking plenty of clean water throughout the day. Proper hydration supports kidney function and helps flush out toxins.
3. **Herbal Cleanses:** Incorporate herbs known for their detoxifying properties, such as milk thistle, dandelion root, and burdock. These herbs support liver function and help remove toxins from the body.
4. **Fasting and Juicing:** Short-term fasting or juice cleanses can give the digestive system a break and support the body's natural detox processes. Always approach fasting with caution and consult a healthcare provider.
5. **Sweating:** Engage in activities that promote sweating, such as exercise, saunas, or hot baths. Sweating helps eliminate toxins through the skin.
6. **Dry Brushing:** This technique involves brushing the skin with a natural bristle brush to stimulate lymphatic drainage and promote the removal of toxins.
7. **Probiotics:** Support gut health by incorporating probiotics into your diet. Probiotics help balance intestinal bacteria and improve digestive function.
8. **Epsom Salt Baths:** Soaking in Epsom salt baths can aid in detoxification by drawing out toxins through the skin. The magnesium in Epsom salts also helps relax muscles and reduce stress.

Colon Cleansing Techniques:

1. **Dietary Fiber:** Increase intake of dietary fiber through fruits, vegetables, and whole grains. Fiber helps promote regular bowel movements and remove waste.
2. **Hydration:** Drink plenty of water to keep the digestive system hydrated and support bowel movements.
3. **Natural Laxatives:** Use natural laxatives like aloe vera juice or senna leaves to relieve constipation and promote cleansing.
4. **Enemas:** Administer enemas using warm water or herbal solutions to cleanse the colon. Coffee enemas, in particular, are known for their liver detoxification benefits.

Guided Detoxification:

Always seek guidance from a qualified holistic practitioner when embarking on a detoxification program. Practitioners can provide personalized advice, monitor progress, and ensure safety throughout the detox process. Additionally, several books offer detailed explanations of these procedures and the many benefits of a clean digestive system.

Final Thoughts on Detoxification:

Detoxifying the body is about more than just cleansing—it's about restoring balance, supporting organ function, and promoting overall health. By adopting holistic detox practices and working with knowledgeable practitioners, you can achieve a cleaner, healthier, and more vibrant life.

CHAPTER 28

Chapter 28: Holistic Wellness and Energy Healing B

Holistic wellness is a unique approach to health that recognizes the interconnection of all aspects of a person. Healing must occur on mental, emotional, spiritual, and physical levels to truly experience freedom from dysfunction and disease. When these components are balanced, health is at its best, dis-ease disappears, and individuals reach their highest potential and fulfill their purpose in life.

Best Practices for Holistic Wellness:

1. **Healthy Eating Habits:** Opt for natural, organic products and avoid processed foods. A diet rich in whole foods supports overall health and well-being.
2. **Regular Exercise:** Incorporate activities like yoga, Pilates, and contemporary Eastern movement techniques to keep the body active and flexible.
3. **Relaxation Techniques:** Utilize relaxation techniques like massage, aromatherapy, and mindfulness to reduce stress and promote relaxation.

4. **Quality Sleep:** Ensure adequate rest to allow the body to restore and repair itself. Establish a regular sleep routine and create a sleep-friendly environment.
5. **Natural and Organic Products:** Use natural and organic medications and supplements prescribed by licensed professionals for a holistic approach to health.
6. **Mind-Body Medicine:** Explore holistic approaches to mental health, such as aromatherapy, yoga breathwork, and creative arts therapy, to enhance the mind-body connection.

Energy Healing Practices:

1. **Reiki:** A form of energy healing where practitioners channel healing energy into the patient's body through their hands. Reiki promotes relaxation, reduces stress, and supports overall healing.
2. **Healing Touch:** This technique uses gentle touch to influence the energy fields surrounding the body. Healing touch aims to restore balance and harmony within the body's energy system.
3. **Acupuncture:** Involves inserting fine needles into specific points on the body to balance energy flow. Acupuncture helps alleviate pain and supports physical and emotional well-being.
4. **Chakra Balancing:** Focuses on aligning and balancing the body's energy centers (chakras) to promote harmony and well-being. Techniques may include meditation, crystals, and visualization exercises.
5. **Sound Healing:** Uses sound vibrations to promote relaxation and healing. Instruments like Tibetan singing bowls,

tuning forks, and gongs are commonly used in sound healing sessions.

Holistic Counseling and Support:

1. **Small Group Counseling:** Provides a supportive environment to discuss and work through issues related to work, romance, parenting, and other life challenges.
2. **Individual Counseling:** Offers personalized guidance to address specific concerns and promote emotional and mental well-being.
3. **Acudetox:** A form of acupuncture focusing on detoxifying the body and enhancing overall health.
4. **Herbal and Nutritional Advice:** Provides guidance on using herbs and nutrition to support health and wellness.
5. **Creative Arts Therapy:** Uses artistic expression to promote emotional healing and self-discovery. Activities like painting, drawing, and music therapy can be powerful therapeutic tools.

Holistic Lifestyle Practices:

- **Meditation and Mindfulness:** Regular meditation practice helps quiet the mind and connect with your inner self. Mindfulness techniques can reduce stress and enhance self-awareness.
- **Bodywork and Movement:** Incorporate bodywork practices such as Tai Chi, Qigong, and yoga to promote flexibility, balance, and physical strength.
- **Holistic Self-Care:** Prioritize self-care practices that nurture the mind, body, and spirit. This includes setting aside time

for relaxation, hobbies, and activities that bring joy and fulfillment.

Final Thoughts on Holistic Wellness:

Embracing holistic wellness means acknowledging and nurturing the interconnectedness of your physical, mental, emotional, and spiritual health. By incorporating these practices into your daily life, you can achieve a harmonious balance, elevate your well-being, and reach your highest potential. Holistic wellness and energy healing provide a comprehensive approach to living a vibrant, healthy life.

CHAPTER 29

Chapter 29: Holistic Living and Ayurveda By Nolan

In The Complete Idiot's Guide to Ayurveda, Dr. Eve Adamson explains that ancient Ayurvedic texts describe people as being created as "gestalts," with a completely integrated body-mind system. One of the first beings in these texts, the healer Atreya, was created alongside herbs that served special functions to restore balance. Adamson speculates that Atreya represented the ideal of human beings embodying perfect health and balance beyond time.

One of the most fundamental aspects of Ayurveda is the belief in the body's ability to heal itself. For example, Dr. Adamson explains that when a person experiences depression, changes in diet and lifestyle, emphasizing how altering daily habits can tip the scale in favor of producing chemicals that positively affect emotions.

Principles of Ayurveda:

1. **Holistic System:** Ayurveda is a comprehensive health and well-being system that addresses both the body and mind. It emphasizes the interconnectedness of physical and psychological well-being.

2. **Self-Healing:** Ayurveda promotes the body's natural ability to heal itself by identifying and addressing imbalances. This involves making dietary and lifestyle changes that support overall health.
3. **Individualized Care:** Understanding your unique body type (dosha) and mental condition is crucial in Ayurveda. Treatments and recommendations are tailored to your specific constitution to ensure optimal benefits.
4. **Professional Guidance:** Consulting with qualified Ayurvedic professionals can help you understand your body and determine the appropriate treatments, supplements, and foods that suit your needs.
5. **Adherence to Prescriptions:** Following Ayurvedic prescriptions, including specific exercises and diets, under prescribed amounts and timings is essential to achieve the desired benefits.

Ayurvedic Concepts:

1. **Doshas:** Ayurveda identifies three primary doshas—Vata, Pitta, and Kapha. These doshas represent different combinations of the five elements (earth, water, fire, air, and ether) and govern various physiological and psychological functions. Understanding your dominant dosha helps tailor your diet, lifestyle, and treatments to maintain balance.
2. **Agni (Digestive Fire):** Agni is the digestive fire responsible for breaking down food and absorbing nutrients. Keeping agni strong is vital for overall health. Poor digestion can lead to imbalances and illness.
3. **Ojas:** Ojas is the essence of vitality and immunity in the body. It is considered the foundation of physical, mental, and emo-

tional well-being. Healthy ojas results from balanced living and proper nourishment.

4. **Prana:** Prana is the life force or vital energy that flows through all living beings. Maintaining the flow of prana is essential for health and vitality. Practices like pranayama (breath control) help regulate prana.

Ayurvedic Practices:

1. **Diet and Nutrition:** Ayurveda emphasizes eating fresh, seasonal, and whole foods. Ayurvedic diets are tailored to balance your dosha and may include specific spices, herbs, and cooking methods to enhance digestion and overall health.
2. **Daily Routines:** Establishing a daily routine (dinacharya) that includes practices like tongue scraping, oil pulling, and dry brushing helps remove toxins and promote balance.
3. **Herbal Remedies:** Ayurveda incorporates various herbs and spices known for their healing properties. Common herbs include turmeric, ashwagandha, tulsi (holy basil), and ginger.
4. **Yoga and Meditation:** These practices support physical and mental balance. Yoga postures (asanas) and meditation techniques are tailored to your dosha to enhance overall well-being.
5. **Detoxification:** Ayurvedic detoxification methods, such as Panchakarma, help eliminate toxins and restore balance. Detoxification may include treatments like oil massages (Abhyanga), herbal steam baths (Swedana), and enemas (Basti).
6. **Lifestyle Adjustments:** Balancing work, rest, and play is crucial in Ayurveda. It encourages a harmonious lifestyle that supports physical, mental, and emotional health.

Final Thoughts on Ayurveda:

Ayurveda offers a holistic approach to health and wellness, emphasizing the importance of balance and self-awareness. By understanding your body and mind, making appropriate lifestyle adjustments, and seeking professional guidance, you can achieve optimal health and well-being. Embracing Ayurvedic principles can help you lead a balanced, harmonious life and reach your highest potential.

CHAPTER 30

Chapter 30: Holistic Nutrition for Optimal Health

The phrase "You are what you eat" has become a well-known fact. Research studies in diverse fields such as aging, digestion, allergies, cardiovascular disease, and skin health reveal the significant role nutrition plays. Despite this, many traditional nutritionists and dietitians often overlook the broader aspects of nutrition. Traditional nutritionists typically focus on food from a narrow perspective, while holistic nutritionists or naturopathic nutritionists take a broader, more comprehensive approach.

Holistic nutritionists study the effects of food on the body, emotions, and mind. They look at the individual and strive to find the most optimal diet tailored to that person, rather than a one-size-fits-all approach. This personalized approach considers genetic makeup and other individual factors to determine the best diet.

Principles of Holistic Nutrition:

1. **Whole Foods:** Emphasize the consumption of whole, unprocessed foods that retain their natural nutrients. Choose

foods in their most natural state to gain the maximum health benefits.

2. **Balanced Diet:** Ensure a balanced diet that includes a variety of fruits, vegetables, lean proteins, whole grains, and healthy fats. Balance is key to providing your body with essential nutrients.
3. **Individualized Plans:** Tailor nutrition plans to individual needs, considering factors like genetics, lifestyle, and health conditions. Personalized plans help address specific health concerns and promote overall well-being.
4. **Mind-Body Connection:** Recognize the connection between food and mental health. Certain foods can affect mood, cognitive function, and emotional well-being.
5. **Natural and Organic:** Opt for natural and organic foods that are free from harmful chemicals, pesticides, and GMOs. These foods support overall health and reduce exposure to toxins.

Holistic Nutrition Strategies:

1. **Detoxification:** Incorporate detoxifying foods and practices to eliminate toxins from the body. Foods like leafy greens, citrus fruits, and cruciferous vegetables support the body's natural detox processes.
2. **Hydration:** Maintain proper hydration by drinking plenty of clean water throughout the day. Adequate hydration supports digestive health, skin health, and overall vitality.
3. **Supplementation:** Use supplements wisely to fill nutritional gaps. Choose high-quality, preservative-free pharmaceutical-grade supplements prescribed by a licensed professional.

4. **Mindful Eating:** Practice mindful eating by paying attention to hunger cues, savoring each bite, and eating slowly. Mindful eating helps improve digestion and prevents overeating.
5. **Probiotics:** Incorporate probiotic-rich foods like yogurt, kefir, sauerkraut, and miso to support gut health and balance intestinal bacteria.

Benefits of Holistic Nutrition:

1. **Improved Digestion:** A diet tailored to your unique needs can enhance digestion and prevent issues like bloating, gas, and indigestion.
2. **Enhanced Immunity:** Proper nutrition supports a strong immune system, reducing the risk of infections and illnesses.
3. **Better Mental Health:** Certain nutrients, such as omega-3 fatty acids, B vitamins, and antioxidants, support brain health and improve mood and cognitive function.
4. **Optimal Weight Management:** Holistic nutrition helps maintain a healthy weight by providing balanced, nutrient-dense foods that support metabolism and reduce cravings.
5. **Increased Energy:** A well-balanced diet provides sustained energy throughout the day, reducing fatigue and improving overall vitality.

Holistic Nutrition Practices:

1. **Cooking at Home:** Preparing meals at home allows you to control ingredients and ensure you are consuming wholesome, nutritious foods.

2. **Meal Planning:** Plan meals ahead of time to include a variety of foods and ensure balanced nutrition. This helps prevent unhealthy eating habits due to lack of time or preparation.
3. **Seasonal Eating:** Choose seasonal produce to get the freshest and most nutrient-dense foods. Seasonal eating also supports local farmers and reduces your carbon footprint.
4. **Mind-Body Practices:** Integrate mind-body practices like yoga, meditation, and deep-breathing exercises to support holistic nutrition. These practices can reduce stress and improve digestion.

Conclusion:

Holistic nutrition emphasizes the importance of individualized, balanced, and natural dietary practices to achieve optimal health. By recognizing the interconnectedness of food, body, mind, and emotions, holistic nutrition provides a comprehensive approach to well-being. Embrace the principles of holistic nutrition to enhance your health, achieve balance, and live a vibrant life.

CHAPTER 31

Chapter 31: Holistic Approaches to Weight Manageme

Being overweight can place extra stress on the bones and increase the likelihood of bone loss. Central obesity, characterized by carrying extra weight around the midsection, is linked to increased bone loss. Keeping your weight within a healthy range for your body type and bone structure is crucial. The factors contributing to weight gain and the difficulty of losing extra pounds are numerous and complex. The question of whether slim people stay that way because they eat whole foods or exercise regularly has a nuanced answer.

A holistic approach to weight management always makes sense. Real health is about more than just the absence of illness, and real beauty is about more than size and appearance. Many of the 'Goddesses' and 'Adonises' gracing fashion magazines and TV screens, with their million-dollar smiles, often struggle internally. They present an external appearance that does not represent the reality of their lives. Yet, society aspires to these cutout images, believing their beauty is real when, in fact, it is often not.

Some diets focus solely on food intake and restrictions, which is not a long-term solution for weight management. It's not enough to be beautiful on the outside; true happiness does not necessarily come from fitting mainstream expectations. Spending excessive emotional energy trying to fit the mainstream picture prevents us from truly experiencing life. Engage in life and live from the inside out.

Principles of Holistic Weight Management:

1. **Balanced Diet:** Focus on a balanced diet that includes a variety of whole, organic foods. Pay attention to nutrient density rather than just calorie count. Whole foods like fruits, vegetables, lean proteins, and whole grains provide essential nutrients for overall health.
2. **Mindful Eating:** Practice mindful eating by paying attention to hunger and fullness cues, savoring each bite, and eating slowly. Mindful eating helps prevent overeating and promotes a healthy relationship with food.
3. **Regular Physical Activity:** Incorporate regular physical activity into your daily routine. Engaging in activities like walking, yoga, strength training, and cardio exercises can help maintain a healthy weight and support bone health.
4. **Emotional Well-being:** Address emotional factors that may contribute to weight gain, such as stress, anxiety, and depression. Holistic practices like mindfulness, meditation, and counseling can help manage emotional well-being.
5. **Adequate Sleep:** Ensure you get enough restful sleep each night. Sleep is essential for overall health and can impact weight management by regulating hormones that control hunger and metabolism.

6. **Hydration:** Stay properly hydrated by drinking plenty of clean water throughout the day. Hydration supports metabolism and overall health.

Holistic Weight Management Strategies:

1. **Detoxification:** Incorporate detoxifying foods and practices to eliminate toxins from the body. Foods like leafy greens, citrus fruits, and cruciferous vegetables support natural detox processes.
2. **Herbal Remedies:** Use herbal remedies known for their weight management benefits, such as green tea, dandelion root, and ginger. These herbs can boost metabolism and support digestion.
3. **Supportive Environment:** Create a supportive environment that encourages healthy habits. Surround yourself with positive influences and seek support from friends, family, or support groups.
4. **Lifestyle Changes:** Make sustainable lifestyle changes that promote overall well-being. This includes reducing stress, practicing self-care, and finding activities that bring joy and fulfillment.
5. **Goal Setting:** Set realistic, achievable goals for weight management. Track progress and celebrate small victories along the way.

The Importance of Inner Beauty:

True beauty comes from within, rooted in self-love, confidence, and a positive outlook on life. Holistic weight management emphasizes living authentically, prioritizing overall health and happiness rather than fitting societal standards. By engaging in life fully and embracing a holistic approach, you can achieve a balanced, healthy, and fulfilling life.

CHAPTER 32

Chapter 32: Holistic Health and Acupuncture By Nol

With the growing acceptance of Eastern or holistic approaches in treating ailments, acupuncture has become an area of interest for many. Whether you're studying alternative practices, working in the medical profession, or simply investigating for yourself, acupuncture offers a unique dimension of holistic healing. It's important to consider acupuncture not as a substitute for Western medicine, but as an excellent tool to treat patients comprehensively and holistically.

Understanding Acupuncture:

Acupuncture is a practice that involves inserting fine needles into specific points on the body to balance energy flow. This energy, known as Qi (pronounced "chee"), flows through pathways called meridians. When the flow of Qi is disrupted, it can lead to health issues. Acupuncture aims to restore the balance of Qi, promoting overall health and well-being.

The Meridian System:

The meridian system is a network of energy pathways that run throughout the body. There are twelve primary meridians, each associated with a specific organ system. Understanding the meridian system is crucial for practicing acupuncture, as it helps identify where needles should be inserted to achieve desired effects.

The Acupuncture Process:

1. **Eastern Viewpoint:** From an Eastern perspective, acupuncture focuses on balancing the body's energy and restoring harmony. It involves identifying patterns of disharmony and using specific points to address these imbalances.
2. **Western Viewpoint:** In Western medicine, acupuncture is often viewed through the lens of neurophysiology. It is believed to stimulate nerves, muscles, and connective tissue, promoting natural healing processes and pain relief.

Knowing Which Points to Use:

Acupuncturists undergo extensive training to learn which points to use for various conditions. They consider the patient's overall health, symptoms, and the underlying imbalances to create a personalized treatment plan. The choice of points can vary based on the practitioner's approach, whether it's traditional Chinese medicine or modern adaptations.

Tools in Acupuncture:

1. **Needles:** The most common tool, fine needles are inserted into specific points on the body. They are typically left in place for 15-30 minutes.
2. **Moxibustion:** This involves burning a herb called moxa near the skin to warm and stimulate acupuncture points. It is often used in conjunction with needles to enhance treatment effects.

3. **Cupping:** This technique uses suction cups placed on the skin to improve blood flow and relieve muscle tension.
4. **Electroacupuncture:** This modern adaptation involves applying a mild electrical current to the needles, enhancing the stimulation of acupuncture points.

Benefits of Acupuncture:

Acupuncture can provide relief for a wide range of health problems, including:

1. **Pain Management:** It can help manage chronic pain conditions such as back pain, arthritis, and migraines.
2. **Stress and Anxiety:** Acupuncture promotes relaxation and can help reduce stress and anxiety levels.
3. **Digestive Issues:** It can address digestive disorders like irritable bowel syndrome (IBS) and constipation.
4. **Sleep Disorders:** Acupuncture can improve sleep quality and address insomnia.
5. **Respiratory Issues:** It can help with conditions like asthma and allergies.
6. **Women's Health:** Acupuncture can support reproductive health, menstrual issues, and menopause symptoms.

Integrating Acupuncture into Holistic Health:

Acupuncture complements other holistic health practices by addressing the body's energy flow and promoting balance. It can be integrated with:

- **Vibrational Therapy:** Combine with sound vibrations to enhance healing effects.

- **Aromatherapy:** Use essential oils to complement acupuncture treatments.
- **Nutritional Therapy:** Support acupuncture with a balanced diet and herbal remedies.
- **Mind-Body Practices:** Integrate with yoga, meditation, and mindfulness to enhance overall wellness.

Final Thoughts on Acupuncture:

Becoming familiar with holistic health and acupuncture helps develop a deeper awareness of the interconnections within our bodies and the world around us. By embracing acupuncture as part of a comprehensive, holistic approach to health, you can achieve balance, relieve ailments, and enhance your overall well-being.

CHAPTER 33

Chapter 33: Holistic Living and Aromatherapy By No

One of our extraordinary capacities is the sense of smell, shared with the animal kingdom. This innate perception of aromas allows us to discern whether food is palatable or poisonous, if a place is clean or dangerous, and can even influence mate selection. This is due to the complex information hidden in thousands of fragrant chemicals produced by plants and flowers. Regardless of culture and environment, we have an adaptive set of odors directly connected to emotions and memories.

When in natural settings—like walking in a pine forest, a mountain valley, or by the sea—the smells give us an immediate sense of wellness, bliss, and freedom. Nature's magic treats us to a unique and beautiful awakening feeling of pleasure, while we inhabit a snug, comfortable energy of the cosmos.

Aromatherapy:

Aromatherapy is the technique of using the aroma of essential oils, distilled from specific plant extracts, to stimulate and influence our perceptions, physiological status, or emotional state. It is a holistic therapy, involving seamless interaction between the physical and subtle self. These essential oils carry the therapeutic potential of plants, giving us access to their healing properties.

Principles of Aromatherapy:

1. **Natural Ingredients:** Essential oils are derived from various parts of plants, including flowers, leaves, bark, and roots. These oils contain the essence of the plant's fragrance and therapeutic properties.
2. **Holistic Approach:** Aromatherapy addresses the whole person, integrating physical, emotional, and spiritual well-being. It works by influencing the limbic system, the brain's center for emotions and memory.
3. **Scent and Health:** Different scents can evoke specific emotions and physiological responses. For example, lavender is known for its calming effects, while peppermint can boost energy and focus.
4. **Safe Usage:** Essential oils must be used safely, as they are highly concentrated. Always dilute essential oils with a carrier oil before applying them to the skin and use them as directed to avoid adverse reactions.

Common Essential Oils and Their Uses:

1. **Lavender:** Known for its calming and relaxing properties. It can help reduce anxiety, improve sleep, and alleviate headaches.
2. **Peppermint:** Energizing and invigorating, peppermint oil can help with mental clarity, relieve muscle pain, and reduce nausea.

3. **Eucalyptus:** Often used for respiratory issues, eucalyptus oil can relieve congestion, soothe sore throats, and enhance breathing.
4. **Tea Tree:** Renowned for its antiseptic and antifungal properties, tea tree oil is useful for treating skin conditions like acne and fungal infections.
5. **Rose:** With its uplifting and mood-enhancing properties, rose oil can help with depression, anxiety, and skin hydration.
6. **Chamomile:** Known for its soothing and calming effects, chamomile oil can help with insomnia, stress, and digestive issues.

Aromatherapy Techniques:

1. **Diffusion:** Using a diffuser to disperse essential oils into the air, allowing you to inhale the therapeutic aroma. Diffusion can create a calming or energizing atmosphere, depending on the oils used.
2. **Topical Application:** Diluting essential oils with a carrier oil (such as jojoba or almond oil) and applying them to the skin. This method can be used for massages, compresses, or skincare routines.
3. **Inhalation:** Adding a few drops of essential oil to a bowl of hot water and inhaling the steam. This technique is particularly useful for respiratory issues and congestion.
4. **Bathing:** Adding essential oils to a warm bath can promote relaxation and soothe sore muscles. Ensure the oils are properly diluted before adding them to the bath.
5. **Compresses:** Applying a cloth soaked in an essential oil solution to the body. Compresses can be warm or cold and are used to relieve pain, inflammation, or congestion.

Holistic Benefits of Aromatherapy:

1. **Stress Reduction:** Essential oils such as lavender and chamomile promote relaxation and reduce stress levels.
2. **Improved Sleep:** Aromatherapy can enhance sleep quality by creating a calming environment with scents like lavender and sandalwood.
3. **Enhanced Mood:** Oils like rose and bergamot can uplift mood and help with depression and anxiety.
4. **Pain Relief:** Essential oils such as peppermint and eucalyptus can alleviate headaches, muscle pain, and joint discomfort.
5. **Skin Health:** Oils like tea tree and chamomile are beneficial for skincare, addressing issues like acne, eczema, and inflammation.

Integrating Aromatherapy into Daily Life:

Incorporating aromatherapy into your daily routine can enhance overall well-being. Create a mindful atmosphere at home by diffusing essential oils, use them in your skincare routine, or add them to your bath to unwind after a long day. Aromatherapy can be a powerful tool in your holistic wellness journey, providing both physical and emotional benefits.

Conclusion:

Aromatherapy is a beautiful and effective holistic therapy that harnesses the therapeutic potential of natural plant extracts. By integrating aromatherapy into your holistic living practices, you can experience increased well-being, balance, and harmony in your life.

CHAPTER 34

Chapter 34: Holistic Wellness and Chiropractic Car

The current "fix it when it's broken" approach of Western healthcare doesn't appeal to many seeking better health. For almost 30 years, the wellness movement in North America has gained acceptance and improved overall health by reducing physical, chemical, mechanical, and emotional stress that can cause pain and disease. Holistic wellness uses a drug-free, compassionate form of hand healing called Chiropractic, which originated over 4,000 years ago. This practice focuses on the body's intelligent life force (nerve system) and its ability to heal itself over a lifetime.

Principles of Chiropractic Care:

1. **Holistic Approach:** Chiropractic care addresses the whole person—mind, body, spirit, emotions, thoughts, and feelings. It recognizes the interconnectedness of all these parts and their impact on health and wellness.
2. **Spinal Health:** Chiropractic care focuses on the spine's health, as it is the critical interface between the body and the

nerve system (life force). Proper spinal alignment is essential for overall health.

3. **Vertebral Subluxation:** Chiropractors identify and correct vertebral subluxations—misalignments that interfere with nerve signals. Adjusting these misalignments restores the body's natural ability to heal itself.
4. **Drug-Free Treatment:** Chiropractic care offers a drug-free approach to health, emphasizing natural healing and reducing reliance on medications.

Benefits of Chiropractic Care:

1. **Pain Relief:** Chiropractic adjustments can relieve chronic pain conditions such as back pain, neck pain, shoulder pain, and hip and leg pain. They address the root cause rather than just alleviating symptoms.
2. **Improved Mobility:** Regular chiropractic care can enhance flexibility and range of motion, allowing individuals to move more freely and comfortably.
3. **Enhanced Nervous System Function:** By correcting subluxations, chiropractic care improves nerve function, supporting overall health and wellness. Proper nerve function is essential for the body's communication and healing processes.
4. **Stress Reduction:** Chiropractic care can help reduce physical and emotional stress by promoting relaxation and balancing the body's systems. This can lead to better mental clarity and emotional well-being.
5. **Boosted Immune System:** Proper spinal alignment and nerve function can support a healthy immune system, reducing the risk of infections and illnesses.

6. **Holistic Wellness:** Chiropractic care encompasses every angle of our many interconnected parts, ultimately contributing to a more fulfilling and satisfying life.

Chiropractic Techniques:

1. **Manual Adjustments:** Chiropractors use their hands to apply controlled force to specific areas of the spine, correcting misalignments and restoring proper function.
2. **Instrument-Assisted Adjustments:** Some chiropractors use specialized instruments to deliver precise adjustments with minimal force.
3. **Soft Tissue Therapy:** Techniques such as massage, myofascial release, and trigger point therapy help relax muscles and improve circulation.
4. **Rehabilitation Exercises:** Chiropractors may recommend exercises to strengthen the muscles supporting the spine and improve overall posture.
5. **Lifestyle Counseling:** Chiropractic care often includes advice on nutrition, exercise, and stress management to support overall health and wellness.

Holistic Integration::

Chiropractic care complements other holistic practices by addressing the body's structural alignment and promoting optimal function. It can be integrated with:

- **Yoga and Stretching:** Incorporate yoga and stretching exercises to maintain flexibility and support spinal health.

- **Nutritional Therapy:** Support chiropractic care with a balanced diet rich in nutrients that promote bone and joint health.
- **Mindfulness and Meditation:** Practices like mindfulness and meditation can enhance the benefits of chiropractic care by reducing stress and promoting relaxation.
- **Massage Therapy:** Regular massages can complement chiropractic adjustments by relieving muscle tension and promoting circulation.

The Importance of Holistic Wellness:

Holistic wellness is about more than just the absence of illness; it's about living a fulfilling and satisfying life. By addressing all interconnected aspects of our being, we can enhance our overall quality of life. Chiropractic care plays a crucial role in this holistic model, offering a natural, compassionate approach to health and wellness.

CHAPTER 35

Chapter 35: Holistic Health and Naturopathy By Nol

Holistic health and naturopathy encompass various practices such as homeopathy, Ayurveda, iridology, naturopathy, and aromatherapy. While each approach differs slightly, they share the same holistic health principles. These practices regard the body as the ultimate healer, a complex interacting system capable of self-repair and self-healing. When the body becomes unwell, it should be supported by providing the right conditions to initiate self-repair and healing. The natural state of the body should always be one of good health and balance. Practices like yoga, aromatherapy, nutrition, and iridology can help bring the body to optimal health levels.

Key Principles of Naturopathy:

1. **Self-Healing:** Naturopathy emphasizes the body's inherent ability to heal itself given the right conditions and support. The role of the naturopathic practitioner is to identify and remove obstacles to healing and support the body's natural processes.

2. **Holistic Approach:** Naturopathy considers all aspects of a person—physical, mental, emotional, and spiritual. It recognizes that health and wellness result from the harmonious interaction of all these components.
3. **Prevention:** A primary focus in naturopathy is preventing illness and promoting health through lifestyle choices, nutrition, and natural remedies.
4. **Individualized Care:** Each person is unique, and naturopathy tailors treatments to meet individual needs, considering various factors like genetics, environment, and lifestyle.
5. **Natural Treatments:** Naturopathy uses natural remedies and therapies to support health, avoiding invasive procedures and pharmaceuticals whenever possible.

Common Naturopathic Practices:

1. **Homeopathy:** This system of medicine uses highly diluted substances to stimulate the body's natural healing processes. It is based on the principle of "like cures like," where a substance that causes symptoms in a healthy person can treat similar symptoms in an ill person.
2. **Ayurveda:** An ancient system of medicine from India, Ayurveda emphasizes balance in the body, mind, and spirit through diet, herbal treatments, and yogic practices.
3. **Iridology:** This diagnostic technique involves examining the iris of the eye to identify health issues and imbalances. It provides insights into a person's overall health and constitution.
4. **Aromatherapy:** The use of essential oils from plants to promote physical and emotional well-being. Aromatherapy can be used through inhalation, topical application, or bath soaks.

5. **Nutrition:** Emphasizing a diet rich in whole, organic foods to maintain proper nutrition and chemical balance. Good nutrition is foundational to preventing health problems and aiding in recovery.

Probiotics and Health:

Probiotics, or beneficial bacteria, play a crucial role in improving health. The main probiotics are strains of Lactobacillus and Bifidobacterium, which support digestion and boost the immune system. Taking regular probiotic supplements can benefit certain medical conditions, such as irritable bowel syndrome (IBS), infectious diarrhea, and some children's allergies.

Nutrition and Wellness:

Good nutrition is a significant contributor to overall wellness. By maintaining a proper diet, our bodies achieve the right chemical balance and can heal more effectively. This synergistic relationship between the body and the food we eat helps keep us healthy and supports our ability to fight illnesses.

Holistic Nutrition Practices:

1. **Balanced Diet:** Focus on balanced meals that include a variety of fruits, vegetables, lean proteins, whole grains, and healthy fats.
2. **Hydration:** Ensure proper hydration by drinking plenty of clean, filtered water throughout the day.
3. **Herbal Supplements:** Incorporate herbal supplements to support health and address specific health concerns. Always consult with a healthcare provider before starting new supplements.

4. **Mindful Eating:** Practice mindful eating by paying attention to hunger cues, savoring each bite, and eating slowly. This approach improves digestion and prevents overeating.

Conclusion:

Naturopathy and holistic health emphasize the body's natural ability to heal and maintain balance. By adopting holistic practices such as homeopathy, Ayurveda, iridology, aromatherapy, and nutrition, individuals can achieve optimal health and well-being. Embracing these principles and practices helps create a harmonious, balanced life, supporting the body's innate healing processes.

CHAPTER 36

Chapter 36: Holistic Practices for Mental Clarity

In the midst of chaos—loud honks, endless decisions, constant chattering, and fleeting moments of silence—maintaining sanity can be a daunting challenge. When feeling overwhelmed, seeking meditation, a peaceful walk, a restful sleep, engaging in work, writing, or talking to someone for guidance can help restore mental clarity. Over time, I realized that these moments signal the need to nourish aspects of mental health, reminding us to take care of ourselves.

The Nature of Mental Wellness:

Mental wellness is a fluctuating state with its share of ups and downs, similar to physical health. Recently, the terminology has shifted from "mental health" to "mental well-being," recognizing the importance of healing rather than just curing. Simple acts like hugging a friend or reaching out to someone can significantly impact our state of mind, especially when feeling mentally strained.

Holistic Practices for Mental Clarity:

1. **Meditation:** Regular meditation practice helps quiet the mind and connect with your inner self. Techniques like guided meditation can provide structure and support, especially for beginners.
2. **Mindful Walks:** Taking a walk in nature can clear the mind and reduce stress. Pay attention to the sights, sounds, and smells around you, immersing yourself in the present moment.
3. **Journaling:** Writing down your thoughts and feelings can help process emotions and gain clarity. Journaling provides a safe space for self-expression and reflection.
4. **Digital Detox:** Take breaks from digital devices to reduce screen fatigue and mental clutter. Engage in activities that don't involve screens, such as reading, crafting, or spending time outdoors.
5. **Mindfulness Practices:** Incorporate mindfulness into your daily routine. Simple exercises like mindful breathing, mindful eating, and body scans can promote mental clarity and calmness.
6. **Yoga and Tai Chi:** These gentle movement practices combine physical activity with mindfulness, enhancing both mental and physical well-being.
7. **Quality Sleep:** Prioritize restful sleep by establishing a regular sleep routine and creating a sleep-friendly environment. Adequate rest is essential for mental clarity and overall health.
8. **Supportive Relationships:** Maintain strong social connections with friends and family. Sharing your experiences and seeking support can lighten the mental load.
9. **Creative Expression:** Engage in creative activities like painting, drawing, music, or dance. Creative expression can provide an outlet for emotions and enhance mental clarity.

10. **Aromatherapy:** Use essential oils like lavender, peppermint, and rosemary to promote relaxation and mental focus. Diffusing these oils or applying them topically can have therapeutic benefits.

Embracing Mental Clarity:

Developing mental clarity involves recognizing when you're feeling overwhelmed and taking proactive steps to nourish your mind. Engage in practices that bring you peace, joy, and a sense of balance. Remember that mental wellness is a journey, not a destination, and it's okay to have off days.

Personal Reflection:

For me, guided meditation sessions have been a powerful tool in achieving mental clarity. Initially, these sessions felt physically uncomfortable, but over time, they brought relaxation and calmness. Engaging in mindful walks and listening to spiritual playlists have also played a significant role in my mental well-being. Reflecting on my spiritual journey and embracing moments of stillness have helped me navigate stress and find inspiration.

Conclusion:

Holistic practices for mental clarity are essential in maintaining a balanced and fulfilling life. By incorporating these practices into your daily routine, you can enhance your mental well-being, reduce stress, and achieve greater clarity in the midst of life's challenges.

CHAPTER 37

Chapter 37: Holistic Approaches to Digestive Healt

Our goal is not only to make eating a pleasure but to ensure that the experience leaves you feeling comfortable and relaxed. Digestive health is crucial for overall well-being, and holistic approaches can provide effective solutions for common digestive issues.

Digestive Comfort Techniques:

1. **Mindful Eating:** Practice mindful eating by paying attention to your food, chewing slowly, and savoring each bite. This helps with better digestion and prevents overeating.
2. **Smaller Meals:** Eating smaller, more frequent meals can reduce the distension of the stomach, making it more efficient in mixing and moving food to the small intestine. This can also help prevent heartburn and other digestive discomforts.
3. **Stay Hydrated:** Drink plenty of water throughout the day to keep the digestive system functioning smoothly. Proper hydration supports the movement of food through the digestive tract.

4. **Stress Management:** Stress can provoke digestive cramping and discomfort. Practice stress reduction techniques like meditation, yoga, and deep-breathing exercises to keep stress levels in check.
5. **Left-Side Sleeping:** If you suffer from heartburn after eating, try lying on your left side in bed. Gravity helps food material drain from the esophagus back into the stomach, preventing heartburn.

Key Practices for Digestive Health:

1. **Probiotics:** Incorporate probiotics into your diet to balance intestinal bacteria and support digestive health. Foods like yogurt, kefir, sauerkraut, and kimchi are rich in probiotics.
2. **Fiber-Rich Diet:** A diet high in fiber supports bowel regularity and prevents constipation. Include fruits, vegetables, whole grains, and legumes in your meals.
3. **Herbal Remedies:** Use herbal remedies like ginger, peppermint, and chamomile to soothe digestive discomfort and improve overall digestion.
4. **Avoid Overeating:** Overeating can put pressure on the digestive system, leading to discomfort and issues like heartburn and cramps. Practice portion control and listen to your body's hunger signals.
5. **Physical Activity:** Regular physical activity supports digestive health by promoting bowel regularity and reducing stress. Activities like walking, yoga, and gentle stretching can be beneficial.

Addressing Specific Digestive Issues:

1. **Managing Heartburn:** Heartburn can be managed by avoiding trigger foods, eating smaller meals, and not lying down immediately after eating. Lying on your left side in bed can also help prevent heartburn.
2. **Bloating and Fullness:** Symptoms like bloating and fullness can be related to spleen function. Practices like mindful eating, avoiding overeating, and incorporating spleen-supportive foods can help.
3. **Diarrhea and Kidney Health:** Diarrhea can sometimes indicate a weakened kidney function. Supporting kidney health through proper hydration, balanced nutrition, and adequate rest can help alleviate symptoms.
4. **Orthodontic and Dental Health:** Proper orthodontic and dental health improves masticatory function, supporting overall digestion. Ensuring proper chewing and oral hygiene is essential.

Holistic Remedies and Techniques:

1. **Herbal Teas:** Drinking herbal teas like peppermint, ginger, and fennel can soothe the digestive system and alleviate discomfort.
2. **Digestive Enzymes:** Taking digestive enzyme supplements can support the breakdown of food and improve nutrient absorption.
3. **Castor Oil Packs:** Applying castor oil packs to the abdomen can promote digestive health and reduce inflammation. This technique involves soaking a cloth in castor oil, placing it on the abdomen, and covering it with a warm compress.

Conclusion:

Holistic approaches to digestive health consider the interconnectedness of physical, mental, and emotional well-being. By adopting mindful eating practices, managing stress, staying hydrated, and incorporating natural remedies, you can achieve optimal digestive health and overall wellness. Embrace these holistic practices to ensure comfort, relaxation, and a healthy digestive system.

CHAPTER 38

Chapter 38: Holistic Wellness and Reflexology By N

Today, holistic wellness is part of the booming alternative medicine movement. Many people are stepping away from conventional medical treatments to explore natural approaches to healing, health, and well-being. By definition, alternative medicine encompasses non-traditional medical practices such as chiropractic medicine, acupuncture, and reflexology. These practices often complement conventional medical treatments.

The holistic movement is growing rapidly, with more people turning to natural methods from the East to supplement the medical advances of the Western world. This shift has led to the creation of new holistic medical facilities, wellness centers, and professional schools specializing in holistic health, wellness, and spa treatments. People who prefer alternative methods now have more options to treat their ailments without relying solely on prescription drugs.

Reflexology:

Reflexology heals by working on the feet. It's a science based on the physiological concept that pressure on nerve endings in the soles and toes releases stress and strain in the body. Properly balancing these nerve endings can facilitate regeneration and recuperation. Nature can restore itself simply by walking and standing barefoot, making contact with the earth. Sleeping solidifies this contact with the earth, further enhancing the connection.

Principles of Reflexology:

1. **Nerve Endings Connection:** Reflexology is based on the idea that specific points on the feet are connected to different organs and systems in the body. Applying pressure to these points stimulates the corresponding body parts.
2. **Stress Relief:** Reflexology helps release stress and tension, promoting relaxation and overall well-being. By reducing stress, the body can function more efficiently and heal itself.
3. **Natural Healing:** Reflexology emphasizes the body's natural ability to heal. Touching and manipulating the feet stimulate blood flow and energy, supporting holistic healing.

Reflexology Techniques:

1. **Palming and Thumbing:** Using the palms and thumbs, a reflexologist applies pressure to specific points on the soles and toes. This technique helps maintain the body's good physical condition by stimulating the related body organs and systems.
2. **Sweeping:** In some cases, reflexologists sweep the soles and toes with their whole hands to provide broad, gentle stimulation.
3. **Walking Barefoot:** Simply walking or standing barefoot can act as a natural form of reflexology, promoting contact with the earth and its healing properties.

Benefits of Reflexology:

1. **Improved Circulation:** Reflexology enhances blood circulation, ensuring that oxygen and nutrients are effectively delivered to all parts of the body.
2. **Pain Relief:** Reflexology can help alleviate pain by stimulating the nerve endings and promoting the release of endorphins.
3. **Relaxation:** Reflexology promotes deep relaxation, reducing stress and anxiety levels.
4. **Enhanced Sleep:** By promoting relaxation and reducing tension, reflexology can improve sleep quality.
5. **Boosted Immune System:** Reflexology supports the immune system by reducing stress and promoting overall well-being.

Integrating Reflexology into Holistic Wellness:

Reflexology complements other holistic practices by addressing the body's energy flow and promoting balance. It can be integrated with:

- **Aromatherapy:** Using essential oils in conjunction with reflexology can enhance relaxation and therapeutic effects.
- **Massage Therapy:** Combining reflexology with massage therapy can provide comprehensive stress relief and muscle relaxation.
- **Yoga and Stretching:** Incorporate yoga and stretching exercises to maintain flexibility and support overall health.
- **Nutritional Therapy:** Support reflexology with a balanced diet rich in nutrients that promote health.

Conclusion:

Reflexology is a valuable addition to holistic wellness, promoting natural healing and balance within the body. By stimulating specific points on the feet, reflexology supports the body's ability to heal itself. Integrating reflexology with other holistic practices can enhance overall well-being and provide a comprehensive approach to health. Embracing reflexology as part of your holistic wellness journey can lead to a healthier, more balanced, and fulfilling life.

CHAPTER 39

Chapter 39: Holistic Living and Feng Shui By Nolan

One of the most intriguing and ancient ways to create balance and harmony in personal spaces is through the principles of Feng Shui. While it might be considered more commercial than other holistic practices, Feng Shui is a widely used method for recreating serenity and well-being within enclosed environments. This ancient Chinese art focuses on the flow of energy (Qi) through living spaces and its impact on physical and mental health.

Principles of Feng Shui:

1. **Energy Flow:** Feng Shui is based on the idea that energy, or Qi, flows through all living organisms and enters through the main door. If the space is cluttered or obstructed, the energy cannot flow properly, leading to physical and mental imbalances.
2. **Living in Harmony with Nature:** Feng Shui encourages living in harmony with nature by incorporating natural elements into the home and workspace. This connection with nature promotes a sense of well-being and balance.

3. **Balancing Environmental Energy:** The practice of Feng Shui involves balancing various environmental energy fields around living quarters and workplaces to create positive and harmonious environments.

Key Elements of Feng Shui:

1. **Clutter-Free Spaces:** Keeping spaces clutter-free is essential for the smooth flow of Qi. Remove unnecessary items and organize your space to promote a sense of calm and clarity.
2. **Natural Light and Air:** Ensure that your space has plenty of natural light and fresh air. Open windows regularly and use light, airy curtains to allow natural light to filter in.
3. **Living Plants:** Incorporate living plants to bring life and energy into your space. Plants like bamboo, jade, and orchids are considered auspicious in Feng Shui.
4. **Water Elements:** Water features, such as fountains or aquariums, symbolize prosperity and flow. Place them strategically to enhance the positive energy in your space.
5. **Mirrors:** Use mirrors to reflect positive energy and light. Be mindful of their placement to avoid reflecting negative energy or clutter.
6. **Colors:** Choose colors that promote harmony and balance. Soft, neutral tones create a calming atmosphere, while bolder colors can energize and uplift.

Feng Shui Techniques:

1. **Bagua Map:** The Bagua map is a tool used in Feng Shui to analyze the energy flow in a space. It is divided into nine areas, each representing different aspects of life, such as health,

wealth, and relationships. Aligning these areas with the layout of your home can help create balance.

2. **Five Elements:** Feng Shui incorporates the five elements—wood, fire, earth, metal, and water. Balancing these elements in your space can enhance the flow of positive energy. For example, wood represents growth and vitality, while metal symbolizes clarity and precision.
3. **Yin and Yang:** Achieving balance between yin (passive) and yang (active) energies is crucial in Feng Shui. Harmonizing these opposing forces can create a peaceful and dynamic environment. For instance, soft lighting and comfortable furniture bring in yin energy, while vibrant colors and active areas like kitchens introduce yang energy.
4. **Furniture Placement:** Arrange furniture in a way that promotes the smooth flow of Qi. Avoid placing furniture in direct alignment with doors and ensure that seating areas have a clear view of the entrance for a sense of security.
5. **Clearing Energy Blockages:** Regularly clear energy blockages by smudging with sage, using essential oils, or ringing bells to cleanse the space and promote positive energy.

Benefits of Feng Shui:

1. **Enhanced Well-Being:** Properly flowing Qi promotes overall health and well-being. A harmonious environment can reduce stress and boost energy levels.
2. **Improved Relationships:** Balancing the energy in your space can foster better relationships and communication with family, friends, and colleagues.

3. **Increased Prosperity:** Applying Feng Shui principles can attract wealth and abundance by enhancing the flow of positive energy.
4. **Greater Productivity:** A well-organized and balanced space can improve focus and productivity, making it easier to achieve goals.

Conclusion:

Feng Shui is a powerful tool in the holistic wellness toolkit, offering a method to create balanced, harmonious environments that support physical, mental, and emotional health. By implementing Feng Shui principles and techniques, you can transform your living and working spaces into sanctuaries of peace and well-being. Embrace Feng Shui as part of your holistic living journey to enhance your overall quality of life.

Chapter 40: Holistic Health and Homeopathy By Nola

Homeopathy is a fascinating branch of holistic health with a unique approach to healing. Its origins can be traced back to the principle of "similia," meaning "like cures like." This method involves using substances that cause symptoms similar to the disease in a healthy person to treat the illness in a sick person. Despite initial skepticism, this approach led to the revival of homeopathy, pioneered by Samuel Hahnemann, a German physician who studied conventional medicine in the late 18th century.

The Birth of Homeopathy:

Samuel Hahnemann observed that while treating diseases with doses of quinine, patients began to exhibit symptoms similar to malaria. To test his hypothesis, he administered quinine to healthy individuals and noted that they developed chills and fever, symptoms characteristic of malaria. This observation led to the concept of using "like for like," forming the foundation of homeopathy known as "Hahnemann's law."

Principles of Homeopathy:

1. **Law of Similars:** This core principle states that a substance causing symptoms in a healthy person can be used to treat similar symptoms in a sick person. Homeopathic remedies aim to stimulate the body's natural healing processes.
2. **Minimum Dose:** Homeopathy uses highly diluted substances to minimize the risk of side effects. The remedies are prepared through a process called potentization, involving repeated dilution and succussion (vigorous shaking).
3. **Holistic Approach:** Homeopathy treats the individual as a whole, considering physical, mental, and emotional aspects. It recognizes that each person's response to illness is unique, and remedies are tailored to the individual's specific symptoms and constitution.
4. **Vital Force:** Homeopathy believes in the concept of a vital force that maintains health and balance in the body. Illness occurs when this vital force is disturbed, and homeopathic remedies aim to restore balance and harmony.

Common Homeopathic Remedies:

1. **Arnica:** Known for its anti-inflammatory and pain-relieving properties, Arnica is used to treat bruises, muscle soreness, and minor injuries.
2. **Belladonna:** Used to treat sudden onset symptoms with intense heat and redness, such as fevers, headaches, and throat infections.
3. **Chamomilla:** Effective for treating irritability, teething pain in children, and colic.
4. **Nux Vomica:** Helps with digestive issues, nausea, and the effects of overindulgence (e.g., hangovers).

5. **Apis Mellifica:** Used to relieve symptoms of swelling, burning, and stinging, often associated with insect bites or allergic reactions.
6. **Pulsatilla:** Helpful for conditions with changeable symptoms and emotional sensitivity, such as menstrual disorders and respiratory infections.

Homeopathic Consultation:

A homeopathic consultation typically involves a thorough review of the patient's medical history, lifestyle, and specific symptoms. The homeopath seeks to understand the patient's unique experience of the illness and may ask detailed questions about physical, emotional, and mental states. Based on this comprehensive assessment, the homeopath selects the most appropriate remedy to stimulate the body's healing response.

Benefits of Homeopathy:

1. **Safety:** Homeopathic remedies are highly diluted, making them safe for most people, including children and pregnant women.
2. **Holistic Treatment:** Homeopathy addresses the root cause of illness rather than just alleviating symptoms, promoting long-term healing and balance.
3. **Personalized Care:** Treatments are tailored to the individual's specific needs, considering their unique symptoms and constitution.
4. **Complementary:** Homeopathy can be used alongside conventional medical treatments, offering a complementary approach to health and wellness.

Integrating Homeopathy into Holistic Health:

Homeopathy can be integrated with other holistic practices to enhance overall well-being. Combining homeopathy with practices like nutrition, herbal remedies, acupuncture, and mindfulness can provide a comprehensive approach to health. Always consult with a qualified homeopath and healthcare provider to ensure safe and effective treatment.

Conclusion:

Homeopathy offers a unique and holistic approach to healing, emphasizing the body's natural ability to restore balance. By understanding the principles of homeopathy and incorporating its remedies into your holistic health practices, you can achieve a more harmonious and balanced life.

CHAPTER 41

Chapter 41: Holistic Approaches to Allergies and I

Living a holistic lifestyle can help fortify the body's natural defenses against colds, allergies, and chronic diseases. Holistic solutions include boosting immunity through adequate sleep, proper nutrition, and addressing the body's negative states. The reflexology chart on page 261 provides guidance on healing hay fever and asthma while others enjoy their chlorophyll intake.

Understanding Allergies and Immunity:

Impurities that enter the body through the skin, respiratory system, or digestive system can cause allergies when the immune system is not strong enough to break them down or eliminate them. Reactions like sneezing, itchy eyes, and rashes indicate that the immune system is attempting to remove toxins but has limited power. People with allergies often have weakened immune systems and may struggle to filter toxic waste from their bodies effectively. Allergies can be exacerbated during spring and fall or when the body is stressed and weak. Stress is often the most debilitating factor affecting the immune system.

Holistic Practices to Boost Immunity:

1. **Proper Nutrition:** Eating a balanced diet rich in fruits, vegetables, whole grains, lean proteins, and healthy fats supports overall health and boosts the immune system. Foods rich in vitamins and antioxidants, such as citrus fruits, berries, and leafy greens, are particularly beneficial.
2. **Adequate Sleep:** Ensure you get enough restful sleep each night. Sleep is essential for the body to repair and regenerate, strengthening the immune system. Aim for 7-9 hours of quality sleep per night.
3. **Stress Management:** Practice stress-reduction techniques like mindfulness, meditation, yoga, and deep-breathing exercises. Reducing stress levels helps maintain a strong immune system.
4. **Regular Exercise:** Engage in regular physical activity to support overall health and enhance immune function. Activities like walking, jogging, yoga, and strength training can be beneficial.
5. **Hydration:** Stay properly hydrated by drinking plenty of clean water throughout the day. Hydration supports the body's natural detoxification processes and helps remove impurities.

Holistic Remedies for Allergies:

1. **Herbal Remedies:** Incorporate herbs known for their immune-boosting properties, such as echinacea, garlic, and elderberry. These herbs can help reduce allergy symptoms and strengthen the immune system.
2. **Probiotics:** Taking probiotic supplements supports gut health and boosts immunity. Foods like yogurt, kefir, sauerkraut, and kimchi are rich in probiotics.

3. **Honey:** Local honey can help desensitize the body to pollen and reduce allergy symptoms. Consuming a small amount of local honey daily can provide relief.
4. **Essential Oils:** Use essential oils like peppermint, lavender, and eucalyptus in diffusers or topically to relieve allergy symptoms and support respiratory health.
5. **Neti Pot:** A neti pot can help clear nasal passages and reduce sinus congestion. Using a saline solution, flush out impurities and allergens from the nasal cavities.

Addressing Allergies Holistically:

1. **Detoxification:** Support the body's natural detoxification processes by consuming detoxifying foods like leafy greens, citrus fruits, and cruciferous vegetables. Herbal teas and detox baths can also aid in removing impurities.
2. **Avoid Triggers:** Identify and avoid allergy triggers, such as certain foods, pollen, dust, and pet dander. Keeping your living environment clean and free of allergens can reduce symptoms.
3. **Air Quality:** Maintain good indoor air quality by using air purifiers, keeping windows open for ventilation, and avoiding the use of harsh chemicals and synthetic fragrances.
4. **Skin Care:** Use natural, hypoallergenic skincare products to avoid irritating the skin. Herbal remedies and essential oils can soothe skin reactions.

Strengthening Immunity:

1. **Vitamin D:** Ensure adequate Vitamin D intake by spending time in sunlight or taking supplements. Vitamin D is essential for immune function and overall health.
2. **Zinc:** Zinc is a mineral that supports immune function. Foods like nuts, seeds, and legumes are good sources of zinc, and supplements can also be beneficial.
3. **Antioxidants:** Consume foods rich in antioxidants, such as berries, nuts, and dark chocolate. Antioxidants help protect the body from oxidative stress and support immune health.
4. **Rest and Relaxation:** Prioritize rest and relaxation to allow the body to recover and strengthen. Regular breaks and leisure activities can reduce stress and enhance immunity.
5. **Hygiene Practices:** Maintain good hygiene practices, such as regular handwashing, to prevent the spread of infections and support a healthy immune system.

Conclusion:

Holistic approaches to allergies and immunity emphasize the importance of a balanced, healthy lifestyle. By incorporating these practices and remedies into your daily routine, you can boost your immune system, reduce allergy symptoms, and achieve overall well-being. Embrace these holistic solutions to lead a healthier life, free from the discomfort of allergies and with a robust immune system.

CHAPTER 42

Chapter 42: Holistic Wellness and Sound Therapy By

Exercise for the body, mind, and spirit is an important pillar of holistic wellness. The universe increasingly recognizes sound therapy as a powerful alternative for transforming physical, emotional, and mental conditions. It's believed that 80% of diseases are caused or affected by our negative emotions, 11% by stress, and only 9% by accidents or lifestyle choices. By effectively allowing and releasing these emotions, holistic wellness and sound therapy can regulate emotional energy, promoting alignment and healing.

Principles of Sound Therapy:

1. **Vibrational Energy:** Sound therapy works on the principle that everything in the universe, including the human body, vibrates at specific frequencies. Sound energy can help align and balance these vibrations, promoting healing.
2. **Healing Through Frequency:** Different sounds and frequencies have unique healing properties. By using specific tones, sound therapy aims to restore harmony and balance to the body's energy fields.

3. **Emotional Release:** Sound therapy allows the release of suppressed emotions, helping to alleviate stress and emotional blockages. This release can lead to improved mental and emotional well-being.
4. **Holistic Approach:** Sound therapy considers the interconnectedness of the body, mind, and spirit. It complements conventional medical treatments and can reduce the need for medication in some cases.

Common Sound Therapy Techniques:

1. **Tuning Forks:** Tuning forks produce specific frequencies that can be applied to different parts of the body. They help align and balance the body's energy fields, promoting physical and emotional healing.
2. **Singing Bowls:** Tibetan singing bowls and crystal bowls are used to create resonant sounds that promote relaxation and meditation. The vibrations from the bowls can help clear energy blockages and support overall wellness.
3. **Gongs:** Gong baths involve playing large gongs to produce deep, resonant sounds. The vibrations from the gongs can induce a state of deep relaxation and facilitate emotional release.
4. **Binaural Beats:** Binaural beats involve playing two slightly different frequencies in each ear. The brain perceives a third frequency, which can influence brainwave activity and promote relaxation, focus, or sleep.
5. **Mantras and Chanting:** Repeating mantras or engaging in chanting can create powerful vibrations that support mental clarity, emotional balance, and spiritual growth.

Benefits of Sound Therapy:

1. **Stress Reduction:** Sound therapy helps reduce stress by promoting relaxation and calming the nervous system. The soothing sounds can lower cortisol levels and reduce anxiety.
2. **Improved Sleep:** By promoting relaxation and reducing stress, sound therapy can improve sleep quality and address insomnia.
3. **Enhanced Mental Clarity:** Sound therapy can enhance mental clarity and focus by balancing brainwave activity. It can improve cognitive function and support mindfulness practices.
4. **Emotional Healing:** Sound therapy allows the release of suppressed emotions, helping to alleviate emotional blockages and promote emotional well-being.
5. **Physical Healing:** The vibrations from sound therapy can support physical healing by improving circulation, reducing pain, and promoting the body's natural healing processes.

Integrating Sound Therapy into Daily Life:

1. **Daily Meditation:** Incorporate sound therapy into your daily meditation practice by using singing bowls, tuning forks, or binaural beats. This can enhance the depth and effectiveness of your meditation.
2. **Relaxation:** Use sound therapy for relaxation by listening to calming music, nature sounds, or guided sound meditations. This can help reduce stress and promote a sense of calm.
3. **Emotional Release:** Engage in sound therapy sessions to release suppressed emotions and support emotional healing. Techniques like gong baths or chanting can be particularly effective.

4. **Sleep Aid:** Use sound therapy as a sleep aid by playing gentle, soothing sounds or binaural beats before bedtime. This can improve sleep quality and help you fall asleep more easily.
5. **Creative Expression:** Explore your creativity by experimenting with different sound therapy techniques. Creating music, chanting, or playing instruments can be a form of artistic expression and emotional release.

Conclusion:

Sound therapy is a powerful tool in holistic wellness, offering a unique approach to healing and balance. By integrating sound therapy into your daily life, you can enhance your physical, emotional, and mental well-being. Embrace the transformative potential of sound therapy to achieve harmony and alignment, leading to a healthier and more fulfilling life.

www.ingramcontent.com/pod-product-compliance
Lightning Source LLC
LaVergne TN
LVHW100316210926
848480LV00003B/1148
* 9 7 9 8 3 4 8 3 8 3 1 9 0 *